The Sensorimotor Performance Analysis

by
Eileen W. Richter, MPH, OTR, FAOTA
and
Patricia C. Montgomery, PhD, PT

PDP Press • Hugo, Minnesota
1989

About the Authors

Eileen Whalin Richter, MPH, OTR, FAOTA, received her degree in occupational therapy from the College of St. Catherine. She has years of pediatric experience in a variety of settings, including children's hospitals, public schools, preschools and neonatal intensive care units. She has extensive background in sensory integration theory and treatment, is NDT certified and has completed the NDT Baby Course. Ms. Richter earned a Masters in Public Health degree from the University of Minnesota specializing in Maternal and Child Health. She has lectured throughout the United States on topics related to sensorimotor integration and pediatric occupational therapy and has promoted continuing professional education among multidisciplinary pediatric personnel through her privately owned organization *Professional Development Programs*. In recognition for her contributions to professional education, Ms. Richter was inducted to the Roster of Fellows of the American Occupational Therapy Association in 1989.

Patricia C. Montgomery, PhD, PT, received a BS in physical therapy from the Univesity of Oklahoma, a MA in educational psychology and a PhD in child psychology from the University of Minnesota. She is currently in private practice in pediatric physical therapy in Minneapolis, Minnesota. Dr. Montgomery has been a physical therapy faculty member at the University of Tennessee, Memphis, Hahnemann University in Philadelphia, and at the University of Minnesota, and a faculty emeritus of Sensory Integration International, Torrence, California. She is actively involved in presenting continuing education workshops for developmental therapists, has done considerable research and published extensively in the area of pediatrics.

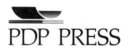

PDP PRESS

Copyright © 1988 by Richter, E.W. & Montgomery, P.C.

First Printing, 1989, by PDP Press
Second Printing, 1991, by PDP Press
Third Printing, 1995, by PDP Press

PDP Press is a subsidiary of
PDP Products, 12015 North July Avenue, Hugo, Minnesota 55038

ISBN No: 0-9623703-1-2

Library of Congress Catalogue No. 88-63896

Table of Contents

Acknowledgment

Grateful appreciation is extended to Jan Kundert, OTR, Mary Rae Freeberg, OTR, Molly McEwen, OTR, Fran Rosen, COTA, and Jan Gauger, PT for their clinical assistance and personal support during the development of the SPA; to Elnora M. Gilfoyle, OTR, FAOTA for her encouragement and advice on preparing the material for dissemination; and to the children of BridgeView School who taught us so much.

The Sensorimotor
Performance Analysis

Introduction

A primary responsibility of occupational and physical therapists working with pediatric populations is planning individualized treatment programs for children and adolescents with various disabilities. Tools are needed both to assess these clients and to provide information about the types of intervention required. The more specific the information these tools provide, the more effectively therapists can plan intervention strategies.

In addition, occupational and physical therapists often perceive, on a subjective basis, that children improve in postural responses and quality of movement following therapeutic intervention. However, few tools objectively document such subtle changes.

Some standardized motor scales simply consider whether or not a child can accomplish a specific skill (Gesell & Armatruda, 1974; Frankenburg, Dodd, & Fandal, 1970). This skill is then correlated to the developmental age at which it normally occurs. Other tests (particularly of fine motor or perceptual motor functions) assess the child's abilities by the number of items he is able to complete and by setting time limits on the completion of certain tasks (Stott, Moyes, & Henderson, 1984; Bruinicks, 1978). Neither method of evaluation attempts to record the quality of performance.

Excellent neurological screening tests (Motti, Sterling, & Spalding, 1978) and standardized diagnostic tests of sensory integrative functions (Ayres, 1972; Miller, 1982) exist, but these are most appropriate for learning disabled children who function at a level adequate enough to understand and perform the tests. Few sensorimotor assessments are appropriate for individuals with severe cognitive impairment. Often test items (such as walking the balance beam) are too difficult, and standardized tests are of little value because developmentally disabled children may demonstrate "spotty" skills. With such children, correlation of test performance to a chronological age level does not mean they actually function like normal children of that age.

Traditional assessments of children's motor and cognitive abilities have been norm-referenced. Norm-referenced tests assess an individual's status in relation to other individuals who have been measured by the same device. Intelligence tests, such as the Stanford-Binet (Terman & Merrill, 1973), are norm-referenced. In a norm-referenced test, items are psychometrically sound and selected to meet certain specifications of difficulty. The administrative procedures are well delineated so that testing and scoring are standardized. Norms are published, and scores are interpreted in relation to the scores of individuals in an appropriate, clearly defined population of which the children may or may not be members (Shaycroft, 1979).

One major limitation of norm-referenced tests, however, is that they do not provide useful information for planning intervention. Knowing how a dysfunctioning child compares to a normative group does not provide the therapist with specific information about the child's maturation level or what therapeutic measures need to be taken to ameliorate the dysfunction.

Criterion-Referenced Assessment

An alternative to norm-referenced testing is criterion-referenced testing, an assessment procedure which is specifically related to the goals of therapeutic intervention (Boehm, 1973). Criterion-referenced tests are designed to assess an individual's status according to some standard of performance. However, unlike norm-referenced tests, scores are interpreted as having some absolute meaning in terms of level of performance or mastery of skill (Shaycroft, 1979). Criterion-referenced tests are more useful for the development of intervention strategies because they define the manner in which the individual — irrespective of others — performs tasks that are closely related to therapeutic objectives. In the case of the SPA, the therapeutic objectives are based on neurological processes rather than specific tasks.

A criterion-referenced test should address a clearly defined domain; for the therapist, this is sensorimotor functioning. Tasks in a criterion-referenced test are specified so that the individual must perform in a certain manner to attain each criterion level: the individual is judged on the basis of these criteria only. The behaviors being assessed are demonstrated through a variety of tasks.

In summary, norm-referenced tests are useful for distinguishing one group of children from another group for placement in special programs or for describing performance in relation to norms for age or grade level. These authors contend that criterion-referenced tests are more useful for assessing the quality of the child's performance on several types of tasks, and the information obtained is directly relevant to planning intervention strategies.

The Sensorimotor Performance Analysis

The *Sensorimotor Performance Analysis* (SPA) was developed in 1975 to analyze movement in a qualitative manner. It has been used in a clinical setting for many years. During that time, multiple revisions have been made based on clinical observations of children's performance of the tasks and the significance of information obtained from each task. From an original battery of ten tasks, the SPA was eventually condensed to seven tasks. These include Rolling, Belly Crawling, Bat the Ball From 3-Point (Four/Three-Point Balance), Kneeling Balance, Pellets in Bottle, Paper and Pencil Task, and Scissor Task. The test items represent those motor skills which most developmentally disabled children (without neuromotor handicaps) can perform or attempt to perform. Scoring is based on differences in *how* the tasks are accomplished (see test forms). Specific criteria

have been defined and are provided for each task (see test criteria). Several of the tasks (e.g. paper and pencil task and crawling) are common developmental test items which should be familiar to those children who are experienced in the school setting. Other tasks (e.g. Kneeling Balance and Three-Point Balance) may be unfamiliar. These tasks are simple but will challenge adaptive abilities.

The primary focus of this analysis is the underlying sensorimotor components of performance. This includes determining the persistence of primitive postural mechanisms. Information is also obtained about sensory processing, developmental lags, postural muscle tone, and bilateral integration problems (including extremity disregard, bilateral coordination, and midline dysfunction).

The SPA is not a diagnostic tool. Although it can be used as a screening device, poor performance should not be interpreted as indicating a specific diagnosis, such as a learning disability or cerebral palsy. The SPA is most appropriately used as a pre- and post-testing device. As a pre-test, the SPA identifies problem areas which assist the therapist in treatment planning, and as a post-test, it measures change following intervention.

The SPA is not standardized or correlated to chronological age. It was developed for educable, trainable, and profoundly retarded children, adolescents, and young adults aged five to 21 years who cannot be tested adequately with standardized tests and who perform new motor tasks slowly. The test can be administered to preschool children, although the Pencil and Paper Task and the Scissor Tasks may be omitted. The SPA has also been used successfully with the adult developmentally delayed population.

In addition to reflecting changes in motor skill, a qualitative analysis of movement aids the therapist in identifying specific objectives for treatment. However, the therapist must be careful to distinguish between therapeutic activities and mere practice of isolated skills. Rolling is an excellent therapeutic activity which can be used in a variety of ways to facilitate or inhibit specific movement patterns. Rolling up an incline, for example, will facilitate a body righting response (Montgomery & Richter, 1977). The act of rolling, however, is not necessarily a primary objective.

The SPA should be considered a flexible tool, and the subjective nature of the scoring should be noted by the therapist when reporting results.

References

Ayres, A. J. (1972). *Southern California sensory integration tests*. Los Angeles: Western Psychological Services.

Boehm, A. (1973). Criterion-referenced assessment for the teacher. *Teachers College Record, 78*, 117-126.

Bruinicks, R. (1978). *Bruininks-Oseretsky test of motor proficiency*. Circle Pines, MN: American Guidance Service.

Frankenburg, W. K., Dodd, J. B., & Fandal, A. W. (1970). *The Denver developmental screening test*. Denver, CO: University of Colorado Medical Center.

Gesell, A., & Armatruda, C. S. (1974). *Developmental diagnosis* (3rd ed.). New York: Paul B. Hoeber.

Miller, L. J. (1982). *Miller assessment for preschoolers*. Littleton, CO: The Foundation for Knowledge in Development.

Montgomery, P. C., & Richter, E. W. (2nd Edition, 1989). *Sensorimotor integration for developmentally disabled children: A handbook*. Los Angeles: Western Psychological Services.

Motti, M., Sterling, H. M., & Spalding, N. V. (1978). *Quick neurological screening test*. Navato, CA: Academic Therapy Publications.

Shaycoft, M F. (1979). *Handbook of criterion-referenced testing: Development, evaluation and use*. New York: Garland STPM Press.

Stott, D. H., Moyes, F. A., & Henderson, S. E. (1984). *Test of motor impairment*. Guelph, Canada: Brook Educational Publishing LTD.

Terman, L. H., & Merrill, M A. (1973). *Stanford-Binet intelligence scale*. Boston: Houghton Mifflin Co.

Theoretical Framework

The rationale for using a sensorimotor approach to assessment and treatment of individuals with developmental disabilities may be helpful for therapists interested in using the SPA. Because occupational and physical therapists should have an extensive knowledge of sensorimotor theory, only a brief review of major theoretical principles is presented (see Appendix A). This review is *not* an attempt to define a new model of treatment. Instead, it will highlight the neurophysiological foundations which led to the development of the SPA.

In the context of the SPA, the working definition of "sensorimotor approach" refers to an eclectic use of neurophysiologically-based theories from such contributors as Rood, Ayres, Bobath, and Grady and Gilfoyle. These theorists have recognized the interdependence of sensory and motor components in normal human development and functioning and in the treatment of dysfunction. The term "sensorimotor" should not be confused with "sensory integration," which in the context of intervention approaches, refers specifically to the theory and treatment principles developed and studied by A. Jean Ayres, Ph.D (1980, 1981, 1983).

Sensorimotor Development and Learning

A basic construct supporting sensorimotor treatment approaches can be traced to early studies in human development by the Swiss psychologist, Jean Piaget (Wurster, 1974). Through observation of infant behavior, Piaget concluded that concrete action precedes the use of intellect and that sensorimotor experiences provide the foundation of mental development. Research over the last 50 years has tended to support Piaget's findings, and other authors have expanded upon his ideas (Gilfoyle, Grady & Moore, 1981). The premise that learning is based on early sensorimotor experience provides a link between sensorimotor therapy and educational goals. Children with learning problems frequently demonstrate sensorimotor problems, and therapists emphasize sensorimotor approaches even in the educational environment. Although, as Ayres has stressed, learning is a function of the brain, (Ayres, 1983) educators rarely receive training in neurology and brain function. In this regard, occupational and physical therapists can be of unique assistance to educators.

Normal Development: Its Role in Treatment

As therapists and other researchers study the process of normal development, it becomes evident that nothing in this process is insignificant. Each development (action/reaction/change) is influenced by previous experiences and provides some component for future development. In *Children Adapt*, (Gilfoyle et al, 1981) outlined a developmental model they designated a "spiraling continuum of spatiotemporal adaptation."

> The spiraling continuum illustrates the ongoing process of development while the spiral-effect emphasizes the integration of the old with the new. The spiraling process of spatiotemporal adaptation has a developmental sequence and matures as a result of environmental experiences and modification of the maturing nervous system to eventually encompass the highest level of complex functioning. The process of adapting lower level primitive patterns of posture and movement to higher level complex skills is the framework of the spatiotemporal adaptation theory (p. 48-49).

In her 1983 monograph *Components of Normal Movement During the First Year of Life* (1983), Bly outlined the same process from a different perspective as she described the components of normal motor development in kinesiological terms. She identified the manner in which the infant moves by muscle activation through elongation and weight shift. The process of developing motor control, although dependent on central nervous system (CNS) maturation and genetically predetermined, is also influenced by environmental experience and provides a foundation for future functional movement. Bly emphasized the importance of balance between muscle groups (flexors/extensors) in relation to gravity and between stability/mobility patterns for proximal and distal control.

The normal developmental process is an integral part of CNS maturation and also facilitates CNS maturation. Therefore, disruption in CNS maturation can result in disruptions in development, and anything that retards development may adversely affect CNS maturation. This is an important concept when evaluating developmentally disabled individuals and is a consideration in designing treatment to ameliorate developmental delays. Activities in which normal children and babies engage provide environmental experiences which contribute to CNS maturation. Normal developmental activities also furnish a model which the skilled therapist follows to involve the dysfunctioning child in therapy. Such activities are rich in sensory input and feedback, but not overly demanding in terms of motor output (adaptive response). Analyses of simple developmental tasks reveal a wealth of therapeutic value. For example, prone-on-elbows control develops spontaneously in normal infants between the age of 3-4 months. It occurs as a result of increasing control (balance) of neck and upper trunk flexion with extension for head stability in prone. At this point, the baby's weight has shifted back, freeing the arms to come forward for weight bearing. While the baby (or dysfunctioning individual) plays and maneuvers in this position, the following sensorimotor experiences are likely to occur:

• Ventral (trunk flexor) muscles are elongated while trunk extensors are exercised and strengthened.

• Weight bearing on elbows provides proprioceptive input to the shoulder joints for stability, while shoulder fixators are strengthened for control of reaching (this provides the underlying postural basis for developing hand use).

• Weight shift on the elbows also gives asymmetrical tactile and proprioceptive input to the surfaces of the forearms, and increases awareness of the hands and arms while decreasing the influence of the grasp reflex, facilitating opening of the hand.

• Equilibrium reactions in the upper part of the body are stimulated by movement and weight shift.

• Increased leg and hip extension result in elongation of hip flexors.

Other therapeutic goals can also be accomplished by carefully adapting developmental tasks. For a brief overview of some of the significant aspects of selected early stages of development refer to Appendix B, "Developmental Milestones and Their Significance." Extensive knowledge of normal development is encouraged (see Appendix C, a bibliography of "Developmental Issues"). In-depth understanding of normal development is critical in both assessing developmental dysfunction and in planning intervention to facilitate normal sensorimotor processing and development. Many authors support the notion of developmental sequencing as an appropriate approach to sensorimotor dysfunction (Ayres, 1974; Bobath, 1967; Gilfoyle et al, 1981; Montgomery & Richter, 1977b; Scherzer & Tscharnuter, 1982; Stockmeyer, 1967), and a number of studies support the efficacy of this model (Barrera et al, 1976; Montgomery & Richter, 1977a; Ottenbacher, Biocca & Decremer, 1986; Weeks, 1979).

Subcortical Function

A traditional model of CNS function describes a hierarchy of reflexes controlled at the highest level by voluntary action. This approach is probably the outgrowth of early studies describing stereotyped reflexes in decerebrate animals and brain-injured humans. Bobath (1985) stated that it was a mistake to apply observations from animal experiments to humans, and in the Neuro-Developmental Treatment (NDT) approach, classical reflex testing has been abandoned in favor of testing for individual reactions or patterns of hypertonus and their influence on normal activity. Refer to Appendix D for a review of the literature on topics related to reflexes/postural responses. The authors' interpretation of differences between classical reflex testing and functional influences of postural responses is outlined in Table 1.

The hierarchial reflex approach contributed to the concept of a CNS that functions primarily in response to sensory stimuli. A new concept also considers the CNS an active agent in the creation and control of body actions through the use of motor patterns which may be activated either by sensory stimuli or by internal processes within the CNS (Van Sant, 1987). For example, the ideation which precedes a motor planned and executed task is internally generated.

Subcortical and cortical processes are intertwined through feedback loops within the CNS. Feedback loops also weaken the concept of hierarchial control (Van Sant, 1987). A *distributed control* model, in which the CNS unit with the most relevant information about the task at hand assumes control, reflects newer information about CNS functioning.

Changing our focus from a CNS as a passive agent responding to sensory stimuli to a CNS as an active agent which can anticipate, plan, and initiate activity (Van Sant, 1987) does not alter the importance of subcortical functions in CNS development and maturation. Sensorimotor development has been thought to begin prior to the development of cognition, and neurologically at precognitive levels of the CNS. Sensorimotor development is facilitated and generalized to other functions through subcortical learning rather than through cortical learning (Huss, 1971; Moore, 1973; Stockmeyer, 1967). Sensorimotor treatment approaches attempt to address problems which are manifest in subcortical structures or functions.

Such problems might include the following:
- Attentional deficits
- Sensory hypersensitivities (tactile defensiveness, gravitational insecurity)
- Poor sensory processing leading to sensory-seeking behaviors, developmental dyspraxia, poor postural control, inadequate response to

gravity (lack of anti-gravity control, decreased righting, and equilibrium reactions)
- Abnormal muscle tone
- Poor integration of primitive motor patterns
- Motor incoordination
- Poor ocular control
- Delayed oral-motor development.

Although sensorimotor approaches are designed to bring about changes in brain stem mechanisms, the influence on and interaction with cognitive functions through feedback loops and a distributed control model of CNS function should also be considered. However, if an individual exhibits problems indicative of primarily cortical dysfunction then another treatment approach may be more appropriate. For example, Ayres (1976) found that learning disabled children who demonstrated prolonged post-rotatory nystagmus following spinning did not respond well to SI treatment. She hypothesized that the prolonged nystagmus indicated a lack of *cortical* inhibition and that these children's problems were therefore not greatly influenced by treatment directed at lower centers. Children demonstrating a *hyporesponsive* post-rotatory nystagmus to the same stimulation made the greatest gains following SI treatment. The depressed response was hypothesized to be related to over-inhibition of the vestibular nuclei or inadequate sensory processing at the brain stem level.

A list of recommended readings on the neurophysiological foundations of brain stem functions and theoretical basis for a subcortical approach is provided in Appendix A.

Sensory Processing

Although newer models of CNS function stress spontaneous (internal) activation of motor programs, neurological evidence supports the importance of sensory input to the developing/functioning CNS. There are approximately five times as many neurons in the nervous system devoted to receiving/organizing sensory information as there are motor neurons (Ayres, 1968). Clearly, the nervous system is structurally designed to make the most of sensory experience from both the environment and through feedback mechanisms.

Animal studies have demonstrated that enriched sensory environments result in a heavier cerebral cortex and increased neurotransmitters (Rosenweig, 1976). Neuroscientists have documented that interaction with the environment has positive effects on the structure, chemistry, and functioning of the CNS. Sensory impulses bring about biochemical changes in the brain which are critical to learning. The nature vs. nuture controversy still exists and has been the subject of a number of classic studies (Greenough, 1973). However, most researchers would agree that the *interaction* of genetic and environmental factors determines developmental outcome.

The effects of sensory deprivation have been studied extensively since the early part of the century. Scientists have been interested in normal human adults as well as infants and children. Ashley Montague (1971) provided an overview of this research in the book, *Touching: The Human Significance of the Skin.*. Much of the research relates to studies of institutionalized babies during times of war. Many of the infants either failed to grow and develop or mysteriously died in spite of adequate food, clothing, and shelter. Extensive study of these cases revealed the importance of *mothering* in normal development. Mothering was defined as loving, cuddling, or handling by a consistent caretaker. Indeed, recent research supports the notion that an infant needs one significant individual to trust and depend on in order to develop normally (Klaus & Kennell, 1976).

Elements of mothering have been studied and have been found to consist of extensive sensory input. The Harlows' (1962) classic studies with infant monkeys determined the importance of tactile sensation to the developing infant. He provided the baby monkeys with surrogate mothers, some made of wire and some made of terrycloth to control for tactile input. Harlow found that baby monkeys with terrycloth surrogates developed better than the baby monkeys with wire surrogates. However, all the infant monkeys developed abnormally. Mason and Berkson (1975) reproduced the study, this time controlling for vestibular input through movement. The surrogates were bleach bottles covered with fur-like material, which were either stationary or suspended and randomly moving. Again, although the monkeys did not develop normally, infant monkeys with moving surrogates coped significantly better. A film made by Dr. James Prescott at the National Institute of Health entitled *Rock-A-Bye Baby* provides a visual record of the studies as well as the aberrant behaviors of sensory- deprived primates. The similarities in behavior of the sensory-deprived primates to some of our more profoundly developmentally disabled clients is striking.

A number of studies have determined the effects of deprivation on normal adults (college students) placed in a sensory-deprived environment with no opportunity to move. The subjects rapidly became disorganized and disoriented, frequently hallucinating. A similar deterioration is observed in adults who are bedridden for long periods of time and unable to move or care for themselves. This is a particularly serious problem for the elderly because many of the symptoms of sensory deprivation are similar to those of senility. Normal functioning of the brain is dependent on a continual arousal reaction generated in the reticular formation (RAS), which in turn depends on constant sensory information (French, 1957). The amount of sensory input needed to maintain arousal levels or to prevent over-arousal varies from individual to individual. This is one reason why sensory stimulation used as a therapeutic tool must be administered in a careful and systematic manner (see Appendix E).

Treatment

Theorists advocating sensorimotor-based intervention models have relied heavily on normal development, sensory processing, and motor patterns in outlining their specific approaches to assessment and treatment (see Appendix F).

The tactile system is generally considered to be primal and one of the earliest developing parts of the CNS. For this reason, tactile input has been used as a primary source of sensory input for therapeutic intervention. Somatosensory (proprioception and tactile) and vestibular systems also mature early in ontogenetic development. Both systems are considered crucial in the development of motor planning and motor learning. Along with visual input, somatosensory and vestibular experiences are often used in treatment.

The emphasis on sensory input and type of input varies depending on the theoretical framework. For example, Rood's approach is based on autonomic nervous system functioning by assessing the patient's sympathetic vs. parasympathetic state. She relied on studies in neuroanatomy and neurophysiology as a rationale for intervention which uses primarily exteroceptive stimuli, including touch, temperature, vibration, and tapping. Much of her intervention is aimed at influencing the muscle spindle.

Sensory input in a sensory integrative program is designed to allow the child/adolescent to experience multisensory stimuli at a level and intensity at which he can cope, react, and plan appropriately (make an adaptive response). Because SI theory was developed primarily for children/adolescents with learning disabilities (without physical handicaps such as cerebral palsy), intervention strategies and activities are often too difficult for the physically handicapped child. Somatosensory, vestibular, and visual input are emphasized, although auditory and olfactory input are also used.

The Bobaths (1967) developed Neuro-Developmental Treatment for children with cerebral palsy and adults with acquired hemiplegia. Although the emphasis is on patterns of hypertonus and automatic postural reactions, sensory stimulation such as tapping; proprioceptive input through weight-bearing, weight-shifting, and movement; and vestibular input through procedures to elicit righting, equilibrium and protective reactions are incorporated in treatment. The emphasis in NDT is on using sensory input to normalize muscle tone. Although muscle tone is a concept which has been criticized (Milani-Comparetti, 1981), the NDT approach also emphasizes the need to provide "normal" sensorimotor

experiences for optimal development.

In summary, sensorimotor treatment approaches are based on a normal developmental model with varying emphasis on motor patterns and sensory processing. In a previous publication, the authors have outlined an eclectic program of sensorimotor activities which can be used to complement the SPA (Montgomery & Richter, 1977a). However, therapists can adapt the techniques of various other therapists in attempting to ameliorate the problem areas identified by the SPA. A review of the literature regarding various treatment approaches and their efficacy is presented in Appendix F.

Sensorimotor-based treatment is not necessarily appropriate for all dysfunctioning individuals, but must be applied in a discriminating manner to achieve positive results. In addition, the use of cognitive cues and treatment approaches, behavior management programs, and sensorimotor programming need not be mutually exclusive when the needs of the individual are carefully identified.

———————— **References** ————————

Ayres, A. J. (1968). Sensory integration processes and neuropsychological learning disability. *Learning Disabilities*, 41-58.

Ayres, A. J. (1972). *Sensory integration and learning disorders*. Los Angeles: Western Psychological Services.

Ayres, A. J. (1974). *Development of sensory integration theory and practice*. Dubuque, IA: Kendall/Hunt Publishing Co.

Ayres, A. J. (1976). *The effect of sensory integrative therapy on learning disabled children*. Pasadena, CA.: Sensory Integration International.

Barrera, M., Routh, D., Parr, C., Johnson, N., Arendshorst, D., Goolsby, E., & Schroeder, S. (1976). Early intervention with biologically handicapped infants and young children: A preliminary study with each child as his own control. In T. D. Tjossem (Ed.). *Intervention strategies for high risk infants and young children*. (pp. 609-628). Baltimore: University Park Press.

Bly, L. (1983). *Components of normal movement during the first year of life and abnormal motor development*. Chicago: NDT Assn.

Bobath, B. (1967). The very early treatment of cerebral palsy. *Developmental Medicine and Child Neurology, 9*, 373-390.

Bobath, B. (1985). *Abnormal postural reflex activity caused by brain lesions*. (3rd ed.). Rockville, MD: Aspen Publications.

French, J. D. (1957). The reticular formation. *Scientific American, 5*.

Gilfoyle, E., Grady, A., & Moore, J. C. (1981). *Children adapt*. Thorofare, N. J.: Charles B. Slack.

Greenough, W. T. (Ed.) (1973). Part III. Environmental determinants of complex behavior. In *The nature of nurture of behavior: Readings from Scientific American* (pp. 83-136). San Francisco: W. A. Freeman and Co.

Harlow, H. F., & Harlow, M. K. (1962). Social deprivation in monkeys. *Scientific American, 207*, 136-146.

Huss, A. J. (1971). *Sensorimotor treatment approaches*. In H. S. Willard & C. S. Spackman (Eds.). Occupational Therapy (4th ed.). Philadelphia: J. B. Lippincott.

Klaus, M. H., & Kennell, J. H. (1976). *Maternal/infant bonding*. St. Louis, MO: C. V. Mosby.

Mason, W. A., & Berkson, B. (1975). Effects of maternal mobility on the development of rocking and other behaviors in rhesus monkeys: A study with artificial mothers. *Developmental Psychobiology, 8*, 197-211.

Milani-Comparetti, A. (1981). Pattern analysis of normal and abnormal development: The fetus, the newborn, the child. In D. S. Slaton, (Ed.). *Development of movement in infancy* (pp. 1-33). Chapel Hill, N.C.: University of N. C. at Chapel Hill.

Montague, A. (1971). *Touching: The human significance of the skin*. New York: Columbia University Press.

Montgomery, P. C., & Richter, E. (1977). Effect of sensory integrative therapy on the neuromotor development of retarded children. *Physical Therapy, 57*, 799-806.

Montgomery, P. C. & Richter, E. (1977). *Sensorimotor integration for developmentally disabled children: A Handbook*. Los Angeles: Western Psychological Services.

Moore, J. C. (1973). *Concepts from the neurobehavioral sciences*. Dubuque, IA: Kendall/Hunt Publishing Co.

Ottenbacher, K. J., Biocca, Z., DeCremer, G. (1986). Quantitative analysis of the effectiveness of pediatric therapy: Emphasis on the neurodevelopmental approach. *Physical Therapy, 66*, 1095-1101.

Rosenzweig, M. R. (1976). Effects of environment on brain and behavior in animals. In R. J. Reichler & E. Schopler (Eds.). *Psychopathology and child development*. New York: Plenum Press.

Scherzer, A. L., & Tscharnuter, I. (1982). *Early diagnosis and therapy in cerebral palsy*. New York: Marcel Dekker, Inc.

Stockmeyer, S.A. (1967). An interpretation of the approach of Rood to the treatment of neuromuscular dysfunction. *American Journal of Physical Medicine, 46*, 900-907.

VanSant, A. F. (1987). Chapter 1. Concepts of Neural organization and movement. In B. H. Connally & P. C. Montgomery (Eds.). *Therapeutic exercise in developmental disabilities*. Chattanooga, TN: Chattanooga Publishing.

Weeks, Z. R. (1979). Effects of the vestibular system on human development Part 2. Effects of vestibular stimulation on mentally retarded, emotionally disturbed and learning disabled individuals. *American Journal of Occupational Therapy, 33, 7*, 450-457.

Wurster, H. (1974). On the relevancy of Piaget's theory to occupational therapy. *American Journal of Occupational Therapy, 28*, 213-217.

Table 1

Traditional Versus Functional Evaluation of Reflex Integration

Traditional Test Method	Influence On Function	Sample Treatment
Crossed extension Tap adductor muscle bellies or alternately flex and extend LE—elicits extension/adduction of LE.	If primitive lower extremity responses maintained or strong, protective and equilibrium responses delayed.	Facilitate hip abductors and inhibit adductors.
Extensor Thrust Leg flexed, pressure on ball of foot elicits extension. **Flexor Withdrawal** Tactile stimuli to sole of foot results in flexion of LE.	Interferes with controlled lower extremity movement and reciprocation; hyper-sensitivity to tactile input; results in deformities or contractures.	CNS inhibition--graded sensory input, particularly tactile. Positioning to prevent muscle tightness.
Positive Supporting Hold in standing position, bounce on balls of feet, elicits extension of legs.	*Presence:* Interferes with voluntary LE movement and reciprocation for gait.	Break up total extension pattern: reciprocal LE activities--tricycle.
Negative Supporting Same as above, but elicits total flexion of legs.	*Presence:* Interferes with supporting responses in lower extremities.	Grade sensory input; facilitate cocontraction of proximal joints.
Moro Sitting: Drop child back suddenly.	*Presence:* Non-functional extension pattern predominates (UE); interferes with sitting balance, supporting reactions of arms.	Facilitate equilibrium and protective extension.
Startle Sudden stimuli (loud noise, light, movement) produces flexion responses.	Non-functional flexion pattern predominates in response to sensory input.	CNS inhibition followed by gradual introduction of stimuli.
Grasp Reflex With head in mid-position, press with index finger on palmar surface. If present, automatic involuntary grasp occurs.	*Presence:* Interferes with manipulative skills; makes transfer of objects difficult; interferes with voluntary release;	Facilitate finger extension, inhibit flexion, ie., hard objects in palm; coarse tactile stimulation-activities such as flicking wads of paper with fingers.

Avoiding Reaction

Quick withdrawal of hand from stimulus, usually with hyperextension and abduction of fingers.

Presence:

Same problems as above, also results in weak grasp; difficulty holding onto pencil, crayon, etc. May interfere with development of protective response.

Tactile and deep pressure stimulation to palms; squeeze toys; activities on hands and knees.

Associated Movements

Extraneous unnecessary movement will be apparent in gross and fine motor activities.

Presence:

Isolated movement difficult; general increase in muscle tension therefore fatiguing, decreases attention span.

CNS inhibition--followed by unilateral movements--avoid tasks which are too complex for child.

Asymmetrical Tonic Neck

(ATNR) On hands and knees with instructions to keep arms straight, turn head left and right. If present, arm on skull side flexes significantly.

Presence:

May crawl or creep with a homolateral pattern, poor eye-hand (i.e. feeding, writing, drawing); interferes with bilateral activities; may demonstrate abnormal head posture during desk activities.

If severe: Head position in midline during inhibiting activities, roll in barrel. If moderate: Bilateral, symmetrical activities with head to side; 4-point activities with maintained arm support.

Symmetrical Tonic Neck

(STNR) on hands and knees with instructions to keep arms straight, bend head down. If present, arms tend to flex.

Presence:

Movement regulated by head position; poor sitting posture; smooth reciprocal movement difficult, bound by symmetrical patterns, therefore one-handed activities such as cutting, writing, are difficult; homologous creeping; uses STNR to assume quadruped.

Tendency to lean on desk or lay head down on desk.

Rocking on all-fours prone scooter board, balance on hands and toes while looking at feet; isolated movements in various positions to break up symmetrical pattern

Anti-Gravity Extension

(Sometimes termed tonic labyrinthine prone). Child on stomach: Arch back, lift arms, legs and head up in extension. Hold (6 year old). If present, child will not be able to do this.

Presence:

Flexor tone predominates and antigravity movements difficult in prone; interferes with development of head righting and gross motor skills such as rolling, sitting, creeping.

Side-lying to eliminate influence; anti-gravity movements in prone (extension); prone scooter board activities; roll with arms above head

Anti-Gravity Flexion

(Sometimes termed tonic labyrinthine supine). Child on back: Curl up in ball without grasping legs for support. Hold (6 yr. old). If present, child will not be able to do this.

Presence:

Extensor tone predominates and antigravity movements difficult in supine; interferes with rolling and attaining sitting position from supine. In young child, head may be thrown back.

Side-lying to eliminate influence; anti-gravity movements in supine (flexion); supine scooter board activities; supine, playing with feet.

Landau

Prone suspension; extends head, results in extension of trunk and lower extremities.

Absence:

Makes trunk, hip extension difficult.

Presence:

Makes LE reciprocation difficult.

Facilitate: Prone scooter board activities. Inhibit: Break up total extension pattern.

Neck Righting

Turn head to side, body follows as unit.

Presence:

Persistence interferes with development of body righting.

Activities to inhibit neck righting or to facilitate body righting, such as rolling up and down incline, rolling with arms at sides, in barrel; bilateral extremity movements which result in crossing vertical midline.

Body Righting

Ask child to roll, segmentation should be evident. If response absent, child may "log roll."

Absence:

Segmental trunk movement difficult (specifically trunk rotation); limits flexibility in all gross and fine motor skills, loses flexible basis for extremity movements.

Head Righting

Tilt when suspended prone, supine, lateral. If present, head should right to vertical.

Absence:

Inhibits development of balance and protective extension; interferes with visual processing and other sensory input; child may support head with hand when sitting at desk.

Slow tilting activities; balance activities in all positions: prone, supine, sitting, all-fours, kneeling, half-kneeling, and standing

Protective Extension

Invert suddenly: Also test in sitting, kneeling, standing, prone-supine on tilt board. If present, child will extend arms in a protective response to tilt.

Absence:

Increases likelihood of injury; makes child apprehensive about moving in space; child may be rigid, withdrawn, inactive; interferes with shoulder girdle stability and upper extremity functioning (fine motor tasks).

Facilitate protective response: Invert child over inflatables such as a ball; vestibular stimulation; activities such as falling to hands and knees from kneeling.

Equilibrium

Tilt in supine, prone, sitting, kneeling. If present, arms and legs will abduct and extend in protective and righting responses and head and trunk will right to midline.

Absence:

Cannot react fast enough to respond to changes in position; interferes with balance and flexibility; makes child apprehensive about moving in space (gross motor); affects emotional tone (labile); decreases attention span; child has poor postural basis for all fine motor tasks.

Facilitate trunk and head righting, emphasis on slow tilting to allow child to right; begin with basic balance activities (rolling, sidelying) and progress with more difficult tasks; provide opportunities for movement on unstable surfaces and through space.

The Sensorimotor Performance Analysis

Overview

The Sensorimotor Performance Analysis is a criterion-referenced assessment intended to provide a qualitative record of individual performance. It has been found to be most valuable in treatment planning and in assessing change following therapeutic intervention.

The client being assessed is presented with a task. He is allowed to perform the task in whatever manner he is able while the therapist observes his performance. The score sheet breaks down each task into the *performance components* necessary to accomplish the task, enabling the therapist to grade the qualitative aspects of the client's performance. This system allows for consistent recording of the quality of the client's response which can be used for comparison after treatment. Criteria are outlined for the scoring of each performance component and have been designated as *poor, inadequate*, or *optimal* (see *SPA Criteria*, page 95). A point system has been devised to allow for quantitative measurement of sensorimotor performance (see criteria).

The SPA was developed for administration by occupational and physical therapists with 1) an academic background in neurobiology, child development, and theories of assessment and treatment of neurological disorders and 2) clinical pediatric experience in both medical and educational settings. Professionals without this experience will have difficulty administering or interpreting the SPA without the supervision and direction of a pediatric occupational or physical therapist. This recommendation is intended only to prevent misuse and misinterpretation which could be counterproductive to the client.

Although administration of the SPA is dependent on some knowledge of reflex integration and test procedures, the SPA can also be used by therapists with limited experience in pediatrics. The information provided by the SPA will be most valuable when combined with some formal method of making clinical observations.

Prior to administration, the criteria and scoring should be studied so that the therapist does not have to constantly refer to the criteria during testing. Criteria should be reviewed periodically, especially if the test is administered infrequently. Administer the SPA to several normal individuals as practice. When possible, have two therapists evaluate the same individual to ensure reliability of scoring.

When administering each task, the therapist may use whatever verbal or demonstrative clues are necessary to induce the client to attempt the activity. Begin with simple verbal instructions; if that is not sufficient, demonstrate or use tactile-proprioceptive prompting to initiate the task. If demonstration is necessary, be sure to demonstrate the task optimally (for example, with belly crawling use all four extremities in a reciprocal manner). Scoring should begin only when the client is actively and independently engaging in the task.

Primary Advantages of the SPA

1. The SPA gathers comprehensive information which can be directly used in treatment planning.
2. It is quick and easy to administer. With a proficient examiner and a cooperative client, the test can be administered in less than thirty minutes (including reflex testing and clinical observations).
3. The SPA provides a baseline record of the quality of a client's present performance which can be used documenting change.
4. By analyzing task performance in relation to sensorimotor components, the SPA assists the therapist in identifying specific areas of sensorimotor dysfunction.

SPA Tasks

Rolling: Rolling was chosen as a task because it is a simple, early sensorimotor activity that requires integration of primitive tonic neck and labyrinthine righting responses as well as some competence in motor planning. Rolling also provides the therapist with an effective way to observe responses to tactile and vestibular input.

Belly Crawling: Reciprocal coordination of upper and lower extremities, lateral trunk flexibility, motor planning, and anti-gravity postural responses are necessary for adequate performance of this task. Although most infants belly crawl at some point in development, this tends to be a novel and challenging activity for the older developmentally delayed child.

Bat the Ball from Three-Point: The major performance components are eye-hand coordination, bilateral integration such as crossing the midline, and stability-mobility functions in the 3- and 4-point positions. This is also a novel task for most clients, requiring adaptation to the dynamic changes required by the activity.

Kneeling Balance: This task provides an opportunity to observe equilibrium in a novel situation in which it is unlikely that balance as a splinter skill has developed. Hip and trunk stability and flexibility are essential for adequate performance.

Pellets in a Bottle: This is a simple developmental task in which sitting posture and fine motor development can be assessed.

Paper and Pencil Task: Pencil and paper tasks are familiar to the school-age client, but in this assessment, the therapist is observing the underlying elements of the task as well as the developmental aspects. Due to the complexity of the task, most areas of sensorimotor functioning can be evaluated in the adaptive response.

Scissor Task: While many lower-functioning clients will not be able to complete this task, it is particularly useful for evaluating the performance of higher-functioning clients. The therapist will be able to obtain data on bilateral coordination, postural control, motor planning, and eye-hand coordination using a fairly complex yet familiar activity.

Equipment

Minimal equipment is necessary for administration: tape, tilt board, suspended tether ball, pencils, large paper, table and chairs (proper height), scissors, pellets, bottle (from a Denver kit), and a drawing of + and o (both should be 4" in diameter).

Tape: Regular masking tape which is easily removable and which will not harm carpet or vinyl flooring is recommended. It should be wide enough to be visually remarkable (3/4" to 1" wide).

Tilt Board: Tilt boards should be available in any pediatric therapy department since it is commonly used for testing equilibrium responses. The size must be appropriate to the size of the client. An inverted foam rubber hemisphere, such as a "Merry Mountain," has been used with children whose weight does not affect the tiltability of the foam piece. [Merry Mountain is available from Skill Development Equipment Co., 1340 No. Jefferson, Annaheim, CA 92807]

Suspended Tether Ball: Tether balls are usually available in school physical education departments or can be bought inexpensively at local discount department stores. The ball can be suspended from anything that will maintain its weight safely. It must be far enough from walls so that it can swing freely for a client on hands and knees to bat. Balloons may be less threatening to some clients, but they are not recommended for this task since they have a different tactile characteristic and do not provide a predictable arc for eye-tracking or anticipating where to bat.

Pencils: Primary pencils are used most often, but color crayons may be substituted. Regular pencils may be used with those older clients who are familiar with them.

Large Paper: The paper should be large enough so that when the client is drawing from one side of the paper to the other, he must cross the midline of his body.

Table and Chairs: Seating for the table-top tasks (pellets, pencil and paper, and scissors) should be comfortable and appropriate for the height of the client. Feet should reach the floor easily. The table surface should be about mid-chest height.

Scissors: Primary scissors should be used since most school clients are familiar with them.

Pellets/Bottle: Pellets should be non-toxic. Pill-size candy such as "red hots" has worked well. ["Red hots" can be found in the cake-decorating section of the grocery store.] If you do not have a Denver kit bottle available, use a small children's aspirin bottle or one of that approximate size.

+ and o Drawings: Show pre-prepared, large (4" in diameter), easy-to-see drawings of a cross and a circle which the client can reproduce.

Environment: The testing location should have an area of carpeting as well as vinyl flooring for the gross motor tasks. The belly crawling should be done on a smooth surface (use of hallway floors may be necessary for this task if classrooms or therapy areas are completely carpeted). The fine motor tasks take up very little space and usually can be set up easily just about anywhere.

Sensorimotor Performance Analysis

Name _____ **Age** _____

Birthdate _____ **Evaluator** _____

Date of Evaluation _____ **Additional Information** _____

Item A: Rolling

Won't lie down to roll_____ Will not roll _____

		Poor		Optimal
1.	Rolls both directions	1 lt___ rt___	3	5
2.	Motor planning	1 lt___ rt___	3	5
3.	Body righting	1 lt___ rt___	3	5
4.	Head righting a. prone b. supine c. lateral	1 1 1	3 3 3	5 5 5
5.	Asymmetrical tonic neck	1 lt___ rt___	3	5
6.	Antigravity flexion	1	3	5
7.	Antigravity extension a. hips flexed b. knees flexed c. arms flexed	1 ___ ___ ___	3	5
8.	Becomes dizzy	1	3	5

Item B: Belly Crawling

Will not assume or maintain a prone position _____

Will not crawl fast _____

		Poor		Optimal
1.	Motor planning	1	3	5
2.	Hand position a. pulls with forearms not hands b. hands fisted c. fingertips only d. palms only e. uses whole hand to pull	1 ___ ___ ___ ___	3	5
3.	Extremity lag	1 lt___ rt___ UE/LE	3	5
4.	Propulsion-feet & knees push	1	3	5
5.	Antigravity extension	1	3	5
6.	Prone head righting	1	3	5
7.	Upper trunk extension	1	3	5
8.	Lateral trunk movement	1	3	5
9.	Crawling pattern a. homolateral/ATNR b. homologous/STNR c. reciprocal	1 ___ ___	3	5 ___ ___ ___

Notes

_____

_____

_____

_____

_____

Item C: Bat the Ball from Hands and Knees

		Poor		Optimal
1.	Maintains 4-pt. position	1	3	5
2.	Eye tracking	1	3	5
3.	Visual avoiding reaction	1	3	5
4.	Crosses midline visually	1 lt___ rt___	3	5
5.	Crosses midline motorically	1 lt___ rt___	3	5
6.	Head righting	1	3	5
7.	Symmetrical tonic neck	1	3	5
8.	Hand position of support arm a. fisted b. fingertips only c. palms only d. whole hand flat	1 lt___ rt___ lt___ rt___ lt___ rt___ lt___ rt___	3	5
9.	Hand position of hitting arm a. fisted b. fingertips only c. palms only d. whole hand flat	1 lt___ rt___ lt___ rt___ lt___ rt___ lt___ rt___	3	5
10.	Maintains 3-pt. position	1 lt___ rt___	3	5
11.	Asymmetrical tonic neck	1 lt___ rt___	3	5
12.	Shoulder control	1 lt___ rt___	3	5
13.	Eye hand coordination	1 lt___ rt___	3	5

Item D: Kneeling Balance

Will not assume kneeling position_____

		Poor		Optimal
1.	Assumes kneeling	1	3	5
2.	Maintains kneeling position	1	3	5
3.	Hip stability	1	3	5
4.	Tolerates movement	1	3	5
5.	Lateral head righting	1	3	5
6.	Trunk righting	1	3	5
7.	Extremity righting a. upper extremities b. lower extremities	1 lt___ rt___ lt___ rt___	3	5
8.	Protective extension	1 lt___ rt___	3	5
9.	Body rotation	1	3	5
10.	Antigravity extension	1	3	5
11.	Antigravity flexion	1	3	5
12.	Symmetrical tonic neck	1	3	5
13.	Asymmetrical tonic neck	1 lt___ rt___	3	5

Item E: Pellets in Bottle

		Poor		Optimal
1.	Trunk stability	1	3	5
2.	Trunk posture	1	3	5
3.	Head position	1	3	5
	a. mid-position	lt___ rt___		
	b. flexed	1	3	5
	c. extended	1	3	5
4.	Uses unilateral reach	1	3	5
5.	Grasp adequate for age	1	3	5
	a. palmer grasp	___		
	b. superior palmer grasp	___		
	c. lateral pinch	___		
	d. inferior pincer grasp	___		
	e. radial digital grasp	___		
	f. forefinger pinch			___
6.	Mouths or bangs bottle	1	3	5
7.	Avoiding reactions	1	3	5
8.	Puts pellets in bottle	1	3	5
9.	Picks pellets up in sequence	1	3	5
10.	Changes hand at mid-line	1	3	5
11.	Preferred hand _____	1	3	5
12.	Dumps pellets out	1	3	5
13.	Tremor	1	3	5
14.	Associated reactions	1	3	5

Item F: Pencil and Paper Task

		Poor		Optimal
1.	Trunk stability	1	3	5
2.	Trunk posture	1	3	5
3.	Head position	1	3	5
	a. mid-position	lt___ rt___		
	b. flexed	1	3	5
	c. extended	1	3	5
4.	Differentiates ends of pencil	1	3	5
5.	Positions paper to body center	1	3	5
		lt___ rt___		
6.	Stabilizes paper with one hand	1	3	5
7.	Pencil position	1	3	5
	a. gross grasp (fist)	___		
	b. lateral pinch	___		
	c. radial-digital pinch	___		
	d. avoids placing fingertips on pencil	___		
	e. thumb/forefinger opposition, pencil resting on 2nd finger			___
8.	Forearm position	1	3	5
9.	Grip strength	1	3	5
	hypotonic	___		
	hypertonic	___		
10.	Drawing pressure	1	3	5
	excessively heavy	___		
	excessively light	___		
11.	Preferred hand (lt___ rt___)			
	a. switches during testing	1	3	5
	b. draws across body mid-line	1	3	5
		lt___ rt___		
12.	Imitates strokes	1	3	5
	a. vertical			___
	b. circular			___
	c. scribbles	___		
	d. bangs/mouths pencil			
13.	Copies			
	a. circle	1	3	5
	b. cross	1	3	5
14.	Upper extremity movement	1	3	5
	a. primarily shoulder	___		
	b. elbow/forearm	___		
	c. wrist/finger			
15.	Associated movements	1	3	5
16.	Tremor	1	3	5

Item G: Scissor Task

		Poor		Optimal
1.	Trunk stability	1	3	5
2.	Trunk posture	1	3	5
3.	Head position	1	3	5
	a. mid-position	lt___ rt___		
	b. flexed	1	3	5
	c. extended	1	3	5
4.	Shoulder position	1	3	5
5.	Forearm holding paper	1	3	5
	a. pronated	___		
	b. supinated	___		
6.	Hand grip holding paper	1	3	5
	a. hypotonic	___		
	b. hypertonic	___		
7.	Forearm cutting paper	1	3	5
	a. pronated	___		
	b. supinated	___		
8.	Wrist position during cutting	1	3	5
	a. flexion	___		
	b. extension	___		
	c. ulnar deviation	___		
9.	Hand cutting paper	1	3	5
	a. lateral pinch	___		
	b. forefinger pinch	___		
	c. thumb/hand opposition			___
10.	Unused fingers-cutting hand	1	3	5
11.	Visual orienting	1	3	5
12.	Cut is continuous/smooth	1	3	5
13.	Straight line is accurate	1	3	5
14.	Curved line is accurate	1	3	5
15.	Preferred hand lt___ rt___	1	3	5
16.	Tremor	1	3	5
17.	Associated reactions	1	3	5

Comments:

Scoring Profile

Sensorimotor Performance Analysis
Scoring Profile

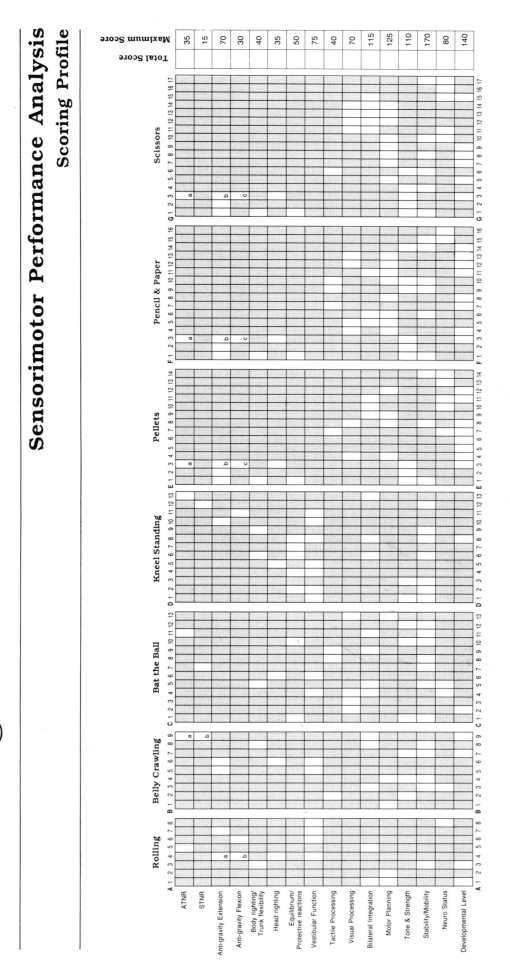

Instructions For Scoring And Interpretation

The Scoring Profile was designed to provide the therapist with a quantitative profile of the client's performance or an overview of the results which suggest patterns of performance and/or dysfunction. Since the SPA provides a record of baseline function, quantification of scores will allow comparison of pre- and post-test results following a therapy program.

Perhaps the most valuable aspect of the SPA is that it provides a basis for treatment planning. The Scoring Profile groups the *performance components* of each test item according to their related *sensorimotor components*. In this way, the therapist can determine major areas of dysfunction and plan treatment accordingly. For example, consistently low scores in motor planning might indicate problems in the area of praxis, particularly if there are corresponding low scores in tactile processing. The Profile is also useful in corroborating the results of reflex testing since many of the *performance components* relate to postural responses (i.e. tonic neck reflexes, righting responses, anti-gravity patterns, etc.).

Scoring Procedures

1. The criteria are scored on the test form on a continuum from 1 to 5. Poor performance is represented by 1, inadequate by 3, and optimal by 5. Study the criteria for each task on the SPA. (See *SPA Criteria* page 95.) If the client's performance falls between the criteria given, assign an intermediate score. Zero (0) represents inability to perform.

2. Transfer the numerical scores from the SPA test form to the corresponding white boxes on the Scoring Profile (see example).

3. If necessary, split the box horizontally to indicate differences in upper (UE) and lower (LE) extremity responses.

4. When appropriate, split the open boxes diagonally to indicate left or right differences. Scores for left should always be placed in the upper left corners and right scores in the bottom right corners (see example A).

5. When a *performance component* is broken into parts, (i.e. A7.- Rolling), the lowest score should be entered in the corresponding open boxes on the Scoring Profile.

6. In open boxes which are lettered to match specific parts of the *performance component* (i.e. anti-gravity extension [a], anti-gravity flexion [b]), only the score for that part is placed in box a or b. The lowest score is placed in the remaining boxes which are not lettered (see example B).

Examples of Scoring

Example A: Performance Component A-1. Rolls Both Directions

On this task, the client rolls only to the left, so his performance is scored 1 (poor) on right, and 5 (optimal) on left. Boxes are marked as shown in the example on page 23. (Refer to Scoring Procedures, number 4, for explanation.)

Example B: Performance component A-4. Head Righting

While rolling, the client rights head in prone (score = 5); does not right head in supine (score = 1); and occasionally rights head in lateral (score = 3). Boxes are marked as shown in the example on page 23. (Refer to Scoring Procedures, number 6, for explanation.)

Determining Total Scores

Total maximum scores for a *sensorimotor component* are based on a client receiving a score of 5 on each *performance component*. When boxes are split, as in left/right scores, use the lowest scores of the two to add scores horizontally for *sensorimotor components*. For example, if a client receives a score of 3 for all 7 boxes representing ATNR, his total score is 21. If he receives a left score of 1 and a right score of 3 on performance component A-4. Head Righting, his total score is 19. When left/right differences are demonstrated repeatedly, note total scores for right and left and take this into consideration when interpreting test results and planning treatment.

Interpretation

Low scores on a *sensorimotor component* are indications of dysfunction in that sensorimotor area. Therapists must use their professional judgment and supplemental diagnostic data (i.e. clinical observations, neurological examination, postural assessment, etc.) to determine whether intervention is required. A small pilot study testing normal 8-12 year-olds demonstrated that scores of 4 and 5 are appropriate. Most children scored 5 on the majority of items. Therefore, when a client consistently scores 4 or less across sensorimotor components, intervention should be considered.

For more specific examples of scoring and interpretation, study the case evaluations provided. All sample activities for the case presentations are from the text *Sensorimotor Integration for Developmentally Disabled Children: A Handbook* (Montgomery & Richter, 2nd Edition, 1989).

Reflex Testing

A short "Reflex Testing Assessment" is included at the end of the SPA form on the case studies. It is designed to be a more formal way of testing postural responses and reflex patterns for comparison with SPA results. "P" is circled when the response is "present"; "F" when the response is "fair"; and "A" when the response is "absent." These scores are arranged to progress from "poor" (on the left) to "optimal" (on the right) to be consistent with the SPA. It should be noted that some responses are optimally "present" and some are optimally "absent." For more information on reflex testing, see the above-mentioned text and Appendix D.

Clinical Observations

Clinical observations provide important information to support and suppliment data gathered on the SPA. The *"Quick Screening"* (page 24) offers the therapist a format for noting observations made in a number of commonly identified areas of neurological function. Scoring and notations made on the form represent the therapist's subjective impressions of the individual's performance and are therefore based on the therapist's experience with and understanding of the processes observed. For that reason, no formal scoring procedures for the *"Quick Screening"* are offered here. Clinical observations are included for all the case studies presented beginning on page 31.

PERFORMANCE COMPONENTS

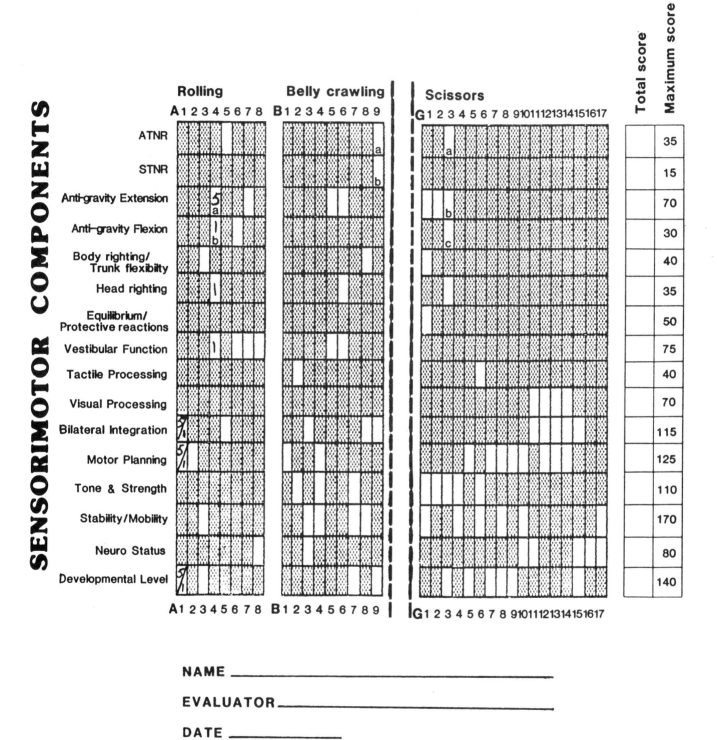

SENSORIMOTOR COMPONENTS

	Rolling	Belly crawling	Scissors	Total score	Maximum score
ATNR					35
STNR					15
Anti-gravity Extension					70
Anti-gravity Flexion					30
Body righting/ Trunk flexibilty					40
Head righting					35
Equilibrium/ Protective reactions					50
Vestibular Function					75
Tactile Processing					40
Visual Processing					70
Bilateral Integration					115
Motor Planning					125
Tone & Strength					110
Stability/Mobility					170
Neuro Status					80
Developmental Level					140

NAME _____

EVALUATOR _____

DATE _____

Eye Tracking: Midline jerk, isolated eye movement poor, visual avoidance, nystagmus

Vertical:

Horizontal:

Convergence:

Thumb-Finger Circles: Sequence, speed, fingertips, accuracy, reverse-pattern, mirroring, intent concentration

Rapid Hand Movement: Speed, accuracy of placement, tone, sequence, asymmetry

Localization of Tactile Stimuli: Estimate distances off

Muscle Tone: Increased, decreased, fluctuating

Distribution: neck/trunk, UE, LE, oral/facial, asymmetrical

Oral Motor Function: Hyper-sensitivity, oral self-stimulation, feeding problems

Sensory Behaviors: Vestibular, proprioceptive, tactile, visual, auditory, gustatory

Precautions:

Psychometric Data

Reliability

The traditional questions of reliability and validity are often raised about criterion-referenced instruments although the appropriate measures for determining them is uncertain (Boehm, 1973). Shaycoft (1979, pg. 60) stated that it is "commonly but erroneously thought, for instance, that standard test theory (including concepts of validity coefficient, reliability coefficients, etc.) is largely inapplicable to criterion-referenced tests." However, if standard test theory is considered in a general context, these factors are applicable to criterion-referenced tests.

A number of methods can be used to determine the reliability of criterion-referenced tests, such as the use of equivalent forms, split-half reliability, and test-retest on the same instrument. Although usually not appropriate for paper-and-pencil tests or for tests measuring cognitive abilities or knowledge, test-retest with the identical form can be used in some motor or sensorimotor tests. A conventional Pearson Product-Moment correlation coefficient can then be computed to compare performance. A criterion-referenced test should be reliable in that measures of performance one day should be similar to measures of performance the following day (the correlation coefficient would be expected to change, however, following intervention or maturation).

Test-Retest Reliability

In a preliminary assessment of reliability, ten trainable mentally retarded children (IQ between 50-80) who did not have accompanying physical disabilities (such as cerebral palsy) were administered the SPA on two separate occasions, one week apart. All subjects were randomly selected for participation in the study with parental consent. The average age of the children (six males, four females) was 104 months (S.D.: 14.5 months). Using the total scores of the sixteen sensorimotor components, the subjects' performance on the SPA was compared to their performance one week later. Test-retest reliability coefficients ranged from .89 to .97.

Interrater Reliability

During the first test session, a second observer simultaneously, but independently, assessed the children's performance on the SPA. Interrater reliabilty coefficients for each sensorimotor component are listed in Table 2. Correlation coefficients ranged from .15 to .91. The data suggest that there was poor agreement between raters on the categories of the asymmetrical tonic neck, the symmetrical tonic neck, and tactile processing. If these three components are excluded, the average interrater reliability for the scale becomes .76. Therapists administering the test should be aware that there may be poor agreement on the three subscales mentioned, and criteria should be discussed in detail to facilitate accurate observation and subsequent agreement.

Performance of Normal Children

The SPA was also administered to ten normal children (five males and five females), whose average age was 111 months (S.D.: 9.8 months). The mean scores and standard deviations are listed in Table 3 along with the scores for the group of retarded children. The relative differences in performance are illustrated in Tables 4 and 5. Test-retest reliability was not computed for the normal subjects as there was a ceiling effect, with normal subjects usually scoring 4 or 5 on every item. Criterion-referenced tests may also be norm-referenced if this is necessary for research or other purposes. Comparison of normative data to the scores obtained by subjects with suspected sensorimotor deficits is essential to establish guidelines for determining when intervention is appropriate.

Validity

Validity refers to how well a test measures what it purports to measure. There are four types of validity: concurrent, predictive, content, and construct (Jackson & Messick, 1967). The first two are considered criterion-oriented validation procedures. The validity to be determined depends on whether the function of the test is to predict future performance (predictive validity) or to assess present status (concurrent validity).

Because the SPA is designed to measure the functioning of children at the time of testing, concurrent validity should be demonstrated. The best way to establish validity is to obtain its correlation with an appropriate external criterion (Shaycroft, 1979). The external criterion should be relevant and uncontaminated by performance on the test being validated, and the reliability of the criterion should be known. Unfortunately, external criterion measures which meet these requirements are not easy to find. This is especially true of a test of sensorimotor functions such as postural development and tactile defensiveness which are neurophysiologic functions, difficult to measure quantitatively, and more variable than motor skills or knowledge in various content areas.

All the trainable mentally retarded children who participated in the pilot study had gross and fine motor delays. However, no specific sensorimotor tests were appropriate to provide an external measure of validity.

Although several years of observing the performance of children with sensorimotor problems on these tasks suggests to the authors that consistently poor performance on the criteria outlined in the SPA is indicative of dysfunction, future validity studies would be appropriate and would add to the psychometric rationale for use of the SPA.

References

Boehm, A. (1973). Criterion-referenced assessment for the teacher. *Teachers College Record, 78,* 117-126.

Jackson, D.N., & Messick, S. (1967). *Problems in human assessment.* New York: McGraw-Hill.

Shaycroft, M.F. (1979). *Handbook of criterion-referenced testing: Development, Evaluation and use.* New York: Garland STPM Press.

Table 2

Inter-Rater Reliability For
Sixteen Sensorimotor Components

Variable	IRR*
Asymmetrical Tonic Neck	.21
Symmetrical Tonic Neck	.15
Anti-Gravity Extension	.86
Anti-Gravity Flexion	.58
Body Righting/Trunk Flexibility	.64
Head Righting	.72
Equilibrium/Protective Reactions	.73
Vestibular Function	.66
Tactile Processing	.31
Visual Processing	.77
Bilateral Integration	.69
Motor Planning	.91
Tone & Strength	.83
Stability/Mobility	.86
Neuro Status	.85
Developmental Level	.79

* Inter-rater reliability

Table 3

Means and Standard Deviations for
Sixteen Sensorimotor Components
Retarded and Normal Subjects

Sensorimotor Component	Retarded Subjects N=10		Normal Subjects N=10	
	Mean	S.D.	Mean	S.D.
Asymmetrical	27	5	33	2
Symmetrical Tonic Neck	10	2	14	1
Anti-Gravity Extension	40	9	62	4
Anti-Gravity Flexion	26	3	29	1
Body Righting/Trunk Flexibility	24	5	36	2
Head Righting	16	5	30	2
Equilibrium/Protective Reactions	38	6	49	1
Vestibular Function	50	6	72	2
Tactile Processing	28	6	37	3
Visual Processing	43	10	68	2
Bilateral Integration	84	10	107	6
Motor Planning	90	16	121	3
Tone & Strength	66	11	98	6
Stability/Mobility	118	10	162	4
Neuro Status	56	9	74	4
Developmental Level	96	13	130	5

Table 4

Mean Scores ± 1 Standard Deviation for Retarded and Normal Subjects on First Eight Sensorimotor Components

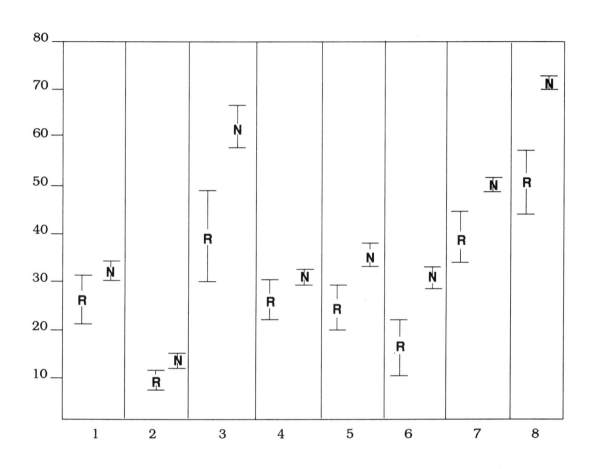

Sensorimotor Components

1 = Asymmetrical Tonic Neck
2 = Symmetrical Tonic Neck
3 = Anti-Gravity Extension
4 = Anti-Gravity Flexion

5 = Body Righting/Trunk Flexibility
6 = Head Righting
7 = Equilibrium/Protective Reaction
8 = Vestibular Function

R = Retarded Subjects
N = Normal Subjects

Table 5

Mean Scores ± 1 Standard Deviation
for Retarded and Normal Subjects
on Final Eight Sensorimotor Components

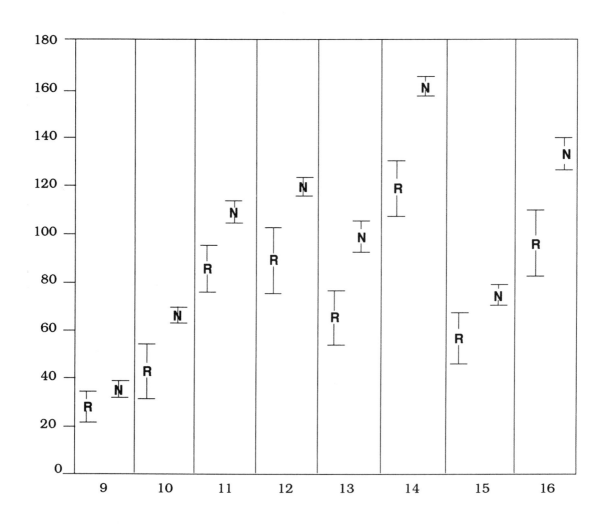

Sensorimotor Components

9 = Tactile Processing 13 = Tone & Strength
10 = Visual Processing 14 = Stability/Mobility
11 = Bilateral Integration 15 = Neuro Status
12 = Motor Planning 16 = Developmental Level

R = Retarded Subjects
N = Normal Subjects

Case Studies

An Adolescent with Profound Retardation

Michael is a 12 year-old, profoundly retarded child who has spent the past six years in a state school for multihandicapped children. He is now in a group home. Michael has no verbal language and limited receptive language, but he has learned one or two Bliss symbols. Although generally hypotonic, he is somewhat rigid when moving and toe walks much of the time.

The primary concerns about Michael are distractability and lack of attending behavior. He avoids eye contact and seems to be in constant motion. He has a seizure disorder which is controlled by medication.

Discussion

Testing and observation indicate that Michael has many significant sensorimotor problems. Like many profoundly retarded clients, Michael's performance becomes poorer as the tasks become more complex (he is totally unable to do Item G, Scissors Task). Academic tasks are clearly beyond his capabilities.

When developing a treatment plan, it is necessary to prioritize the client's needs. The therapist must consider a number of factors. In Michael's case, age and potential for change are major issues. Usually clients in his age group have had many years of therapy, and changes or improvements may have plateaued. However, Michael was in a residential institution and did not have access to an intensive therapeutic program. Therefore, addressing his basic sensorimotor needs in therapy to determine his potential for change will probably be worthwhile.

Another consideration at Michael's age is the demands of the home and school environment. He needs to learn to care for himself and to attend in the classroom. Home and school programs will be placing heavy emphasis on communication and self-care skills. In order to benefit from any of these programs, Michael will have to develop some attending skills.

Michael's difficulty paying attention is probably related to poor sensory processing (see test results). He displays self-stimulating behaviors and excessive movement (wanders aimlessly around the classroom and through the hallways). It will be important to determine whether Michael's self-stimulating behavior indicates that he needs an extensive amount of sensory input to maintain an arousal level or whether his arousal level is too high and he is using self-stimulating behavior to dampen it. In either case, proprioceptive input will be an important modality to use. This is supported by observations that his self-stimulating behaviors tend to be proprioceptive in nature (i.e. toe walking, rolling forearms), indicating his need for that type of sensory input.

Many general therapy objectives have been identified for Michael (see *General Therapy Objectives*). The starred goals indicate the most important needs to be addressed at this time. Although a specific goal statement regarding stability/mobility problems is not noted per se, this is a major deficit area for Michael. It is related to most of the other goals identified and should be addressed throughout most of his therapy activities.

The *Individual Treatment Plan* lists major and specific objectives for Michael's treatment as well as possible treatment activities. These represent a selection and are certainly not all-inclusive. Michael's therapist should determine the appropriate sequence for introducing therapeutic activities since this sample does not necessarily represent choices for the *initial* stages of his therapy program.

Sensorimotor Performance Analysis

Name _Michael_ **Age** _12_
Birthdate _____ **Evaluator** _ER_
Date of Evaluation _3-12-88_ **Additional Information** _____

Item A: Rolling

Won't lie down to roll _____ Will not roll _____

	Poor		Optimal
1. Rolls both directions	1 lt__ rt__	3	(5)
2. Motor planning	(1) lt__ rt__	3	5
3. Body righting	(1) lt__ rt__	3	5
4. Head righting a. prone	(1)	(2) 3	5
b. supine	1	(2) 3	5
c. lateral	(1)	3	5
5. Asymmetrical tonic neck	1 lt__ rt__	3	(5)
6. Antigravity flexion	1	3 (4)	5
7. Antigravity extension a. hips flexed	(1) ✓	3	5
b. knees flexed	✓		
c. arms flexed	✓		
8. Becomes dizzy	1	3	(5)

Item B: Belly Crawling

Will not assume or maintain a prone position _____

Will not crawl fast _____

	Poor		Optimal
1. Motor planning	1	(3)	5
2. Hand position a. pulls with forearms not hands	1	3 (4)	5
b. hands fisted	—		
c. fingertips only	~~4~~		
d. palms only			
e. uses whole hand to pull			4
3. Extremity lag	(1) lt ✓ rt UE (LE)	3	5
4. Propulsion-feet & knees push	1	3	(5)
5. Antigravity extension	1	3 (4)	5
6. Prone head righting	1	3	(5)
7. Upper trunk extension	1	3	(5)
8. Lateral trunk movement	1	3 (4)	5
9. Crawling pattern a. homolateral/ATNR	1	3 (4)	5
b. homologous/STNR	—		5
c. reciprocal	—		5

Notes _____

Item C: Bat the Ball from Hands and Knees

	Poor		Optimal
1. Maintains 4-pt. position	1	(3)	5
2. Eye tracking	1	(3)	5
3. Visual avoiding reaction	1	3 (4)	5
4. Crosses midline visually	(1) lt__ rt__	3	5
5. Crosses midline motorically	1 (2) lt__ rt__	3	5
6. Head righting	1	(3)	5
7. Symmetrical tonic neck	(1)	3	5
8. Hand position of support arm a. fisted	1 lt__ rt__	(3)	5
b. fingertips only	lt ✓ rt ✓		
c. palms only	lt__ rt__		
d. whole hand flat	lt__ rt__		
9. Hand position of hitting arm a. fisted	1 lt__ rt__	3 (4)	5
b. fingertips only	lt__ rt__		
c. palms only	lt__ rt__		
d. whole hand flat	lt ✓ rt ✓		
10. Maintains 3-pt. position	1 lt__ rt__	(3)	5
11. Asymmetrical tonic neck	1 lt__ rt__	3	(5)
12. Shoulder control	1 lt 3 rt 4	3	5
13. Eye hand coordination	1 (2) lt__ rt__	3	5

Item D: Kneeling Balance

Will not assume kneeling position _____

	Poor		Optimal
1. Assumes kneeling	1	(3)	5
2. Maintains kneeling position	1	(3)	5
3. Hip stability	1 (2)	3	5
4. Tolerates movement	1	(3)	5
5. Lateral head righting	1	3 (4)	5
6. Trunk righting	1	3 (4)	5
7. Extremity righting a. upper extremities	1 lt ✓ rt ✓	3 (4)	5
b. lower extremities	lt ✓ rt ✓		
8. Protective extension	1 lt ✓ rt ✓	(3)	5
9. Body rotation	1	3	(5)
10. Antigravity extension	1	3	(5)
11. Antigravity flexion	1	3	(5)
12. Symmetrical tonic neck	1	3 (4)	5
13. Asymmetrical tonic neck	1 lt__ rt__	3	(5)

Item E: Pellets in Bottle

		Poor		Optimal
1.	Trunk stability	1 (2) 3		5
2.	Trunk posture	1 3		(5)
3.	Head position	1 3		(5)
	a. mid-position	lt___ rt___		
	b. flexed	1 3		(5)
	c. extended	1 3		(5)
4.	Uses unilateral reach	1 3		(5)
5.	Grasp adequate for age	(1) 3		5
	a. palmer grasp	___		
	b. superior palmer grasp	___		
	c. lateral pinch			
	d. inferior pincer grasp	✓		
	e. radial digital grasp	___		
	f. forefinger pinch			
6.	Mouths or bangs bottle	1 3		(5)
7.	Avoiding reactions	1 3		(5)
8.	Puts pellets in bottle	1 3		(5)
9.	Picks pellets up in sequence	(1) 3		5
10.	Changes hand at mid-line	(1) 3		5
11.	Preferred hand _____	(1) 3		5
12.	Dumps pellets out	1 3		(5)
13.	Tremor	(1) 3		5
14.	Associated reactions	(1) 3		5

Item F: Pencil and Paper Task

		Poor		Optimal
1.	Trunk stability	1 (2) 3		5
2.	Trunk posture	1 3		(5)
3.	Head position	1 3		(5)
	a. mid-position	lt___ rt___		
	b. flexed	1 3		(5)
	c. extended	1 3		(5)
4.	Differentiates ends of pencil	1 (3)		5
5.	Positions paper to body center	1 3 (4) 5		
		lt___ rt___ *inconsistent*		
6.	Stabilizes paper with one hand	1 3		(5)
7.	Pencil position	(1) 3		5
	a. gross grasp (fist)	✓		
	b. lateral pinch	___		
	c. radial-digital pinch	___		
	d. avoids placing fingertips on pencil			
	e. thumb/forefinger opposition, pencil resting on 2nd finger	___		
8.	Forearm position	1 3		(5)
9.	Grip strength	1 3		(5)
	hypotonic	___		
	hypertonic	___		
10.	Drawing pressure	1 3		(5)
	excessively heavy	___		
	excessively light	___		
11.	Preferred hand (lt___ rt___)			
	a. switches during testing	(1) 3		5
	b. draws across body mid-line	(1) 3		5
		lt___ rt ✓		
12.	Imitates strokes	(1) 3		5
	a. vertical			
	b. circular	___		
	c. scribbles	✓		
	d. bangs/mouths pencil	___		
13.	Copies			
	a. circle	(1) 3		5
	b. cross	(1) 3		5
14.	Upper extremity movement	(1) 3		5
	a. primarily shoulder			
	b. elbow/forearm	✓		
	c. wrist/finger	✓		
15.	Associated movements	(1) 3		5
16.	Tremor	1 (2) 3		5

Item G: Scissor Task

		Poor		Optimal
1.	Trunk stability	1	3	5
2.	Trunk posture	1	3	5
3.	Head position	1	3	5
	a. mid-position	lt___ rt___		
	b. flexed	1	3	5
	c. extended	1	3	5
4.	Shoulder position	1	3	5
5.	Forearm holding paper	1	3	5
	a. pronated			
	b. supinated	___		
6.	Hand grip holding paper	1	3	5
	a. hypotonic			
	b. hypertonic			
7.	Forearm cutting paper	1	3	5
	a. pronated			
	b. supinated	___		
8.	Wrist position during cutting	1	3	5
	a. flexion	___		
	b. extension	___		
	c. ulnar deviation	___		
9.	Hand cutting paper	1	3	5
	a. lateral pinch			
	b. forefinger pinch	___		
	c. thumb/hand opposition			___
10.	Unused fingers-cutting hand	1	3	5
11.	Visual orienting	1	3	5
12.	Cut is continuous/smooth	1	3	5
13.	Straight line is accurate	1	3	5
14.	Curved line is accurate	1	3	5
15.	Preferred hand lt___ rt___	1	3	5
16.	Tremor	1	3	5
17.	Associated reactions	1	3	5

unable to perform (written across items 5–6)

Reflex Activity Assessment

	REFLEX OR RESPONSE	Poor-Optimal		
Spinal	TACTILE DEFENSIVENESS	(P)	F	A
BRAIN STEM	ASYMMETRICAL TONIC NECK-RIGHT	(P)	F	A
	AYMMETRICAL TONIC NECK-LEFT	(P)	F	A
	SYMMETRICAL TONIC NECK	(P)	F	A
	ANTIGRAVITY FLEXION	(P)	F	A
	ANTIGRAVITY EXTENSION	(P)	F	A
	ASSOCIATED REACTIONS	P	(F)	A
MID BRAIN	NECK RIGHTING	P	F	(A)
	BODY RIGHTING	(A)	F	P
	HEAD RIGHTING-PRONE	A	(F)	P
	HEAD RIGHTING-SUPINE	A	F	(P)
AUTO-MATIC	STARTLE	P	F	A
	LANDAU	P	F	A
	PROTECTIVE EXTENSION	A	F ✓	P

	EQUILIBRIUM REACTIONS		RT.	LT.
COR-TICAL	PRONE	HEAD RTG.	A (F) P	A (F) P
	SUPINE	TRUNK RTG.	A F/P	A F/P
(SITTING)		PROTECTIVE EXT.	A (F) P	A (F) P
	KNEELING	EXTREMITIES	A (F) P	A (F) P

Notes

_____
_____
_____
_____
_____
_____

Eye Tracking: Midline jerk, isolated eye movement poor, (visual avoidance) nystagmus

Vertical:

Horizontal: }— *None*

Convergence:

Thumb-Finger Circles: Sequence, speed, (fingertips) accuracy, reverse-pattern, mirroring, intent concentration
— *poor*

Lots of overflow - unable to perform

Rapid Hand Movement: Speed, accuracy of placement, tone, (sequence) asymmetry
floppy   *poor*

Localization of Tactile Stimuli: Estimate distances off

Unable to perform

Muscle Tone: Increased, (decreased) fluctuating
generally

Distribution: neck/trunk, UE, LE (oral/facial) asymmetrical
decreased
mouth open most of time

Oral Motor Function: Hyper-sensitivity, oral self-stimulation, feeding problems

Poor oral motor coordination

Sensory Behaviors: Vestibular, (proprioceptive) tactile (visual) auditory, gustatory
distractible
rolls forearms,
toe walks, etc.

Precautions:

Sensorimotor Performance Analysis
Scoring Profile

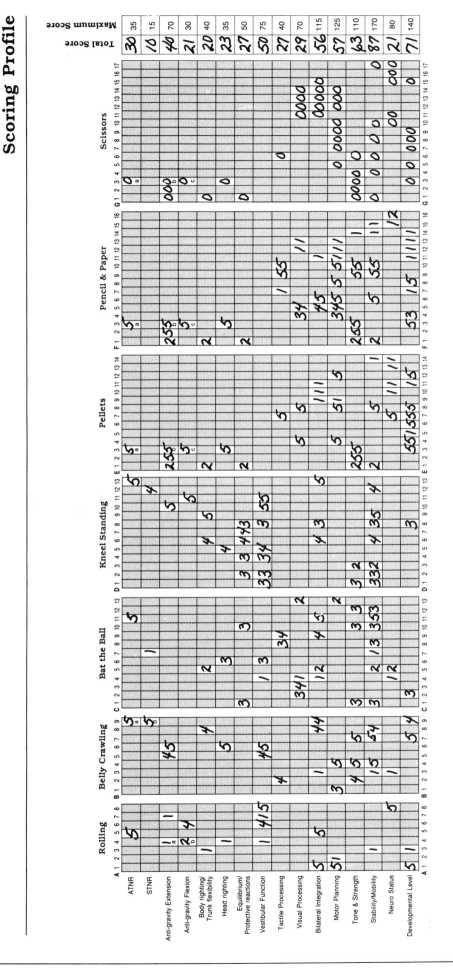

Occupational/Physical Therapy Department
General Therapy Objectives

Name: _Michael_   Therapist(s): _E.R_

Schedule: _____   Date: _01/15/88_

Sensory-Related Goals
     _____ Decrease oversensitivity to sensory stimulation
     _____ Decrease tactile defensiveness
*   _X_ Develop awareness of body in space
     _____ Increase activity level
     _____ Decrease activity level
*   _X_ Decrease self-stimulating activities

Gross Motor Goals
*   _X_ Improve postural control and movement responses (balance)
    _X_ Improve developmental skills
    _X_ Increase strength
    _____ Increase flexibility
    _____ Increase endurance
    _X_ Improve gross motor planning (ability to plan and carry out
        coordinated movement)

Fine Motor Goals
*   _X_ Improve shoulder control
    _____ Develop gross grasp and release
    _X_ Improve hand/finger coordination and manipulation skills
    _X_ Improve bilateral coordination
    _X_ Improve fine motor planning skills
    _X_ Improve daily living skills

Visual Goals
*   _X_ Improve visual focus and attention
    _X_ Improve eye tracking skills
    _X_ Improve eye/hand coordination

Behavioral Goals
*   _X_ Improve attending behaviors
    _X_ Increase group interaction
    _X_ Improve ability to follow directions

Occupational/Physical Therapy
Individual Treatment Plan

Name: _____Michael_____

Age: ____12_____ Rm: _102_____

Teacher: __Mrs. Johnson_____

Precautions: __seizure disorder_____

Therapist: __E.R._____ Date: _01/15/88_____

Major Objectives

1. Decrease self-stimulating behavior.
2. Improve visual focus and attention behavior.
3. Improve postural control (stability/mobility patterns).

Specific Objectives

1. Michael will sit with the teacher or group for 10 minutes without getting up to wander around the classroom.
2. Michael will attend to a sorting task for 2 minutes.
3. Michael will demonstrate some trunk rotation and segmentation of head and trunk during rolling.

Treatment Plan

CNS Preparation: *Decrease self-stimulation while increasing attending/alertness*

• *Bounce on trampoline or therapy ball in sitting position*
• *Swing in hammock in prone position*
• *Push a weighted cart or heavy object*

Sensory Activities: *Tactile/vestibular/proprioceptive*

• *Roll on different surfaces such as carpet, mats, incline*
• *Draw with chalk on carpet; erase with hands*
• *Play "hot dog" (roll up in mat or blanket)*

Oral and Pre-Speech Activities: *Requires further evaluation and planning not covered here.*

Gross Motor Activities: *Begin with simple developmental tasks*

• *Supine activities such as raise and wave arms and legs; hug bolsters/pillows; bat a swinging ball*
• *Prone on elbows activities which stimulate weight shift for reaching*
• *Push heavy objects such as a weighted cart, heavy doors, another child in a barrel*

Fine Motor-Manipulative Activities:

• *Gross grasp-release activities (with upper extremity weight bearing in prone-on-elbows); squeeze objects such as toys, sponges, clay, etc.*
• *Tug-O-War, or pull self back and forth in the hammock using a rope or inner tube rubber*

Visual Skills:

• *Dig for objects hidden in substances of various textures such as popcorn, sand, water, styrofoam pellets, acquarium gravel.*
• *Find body parts such as hands, feet, and arms with a flashlight in the dark*

Behavior: *(See sensory activities)*

A Preschool Child with General Developmental Delays

Lon is a cooperative 3 year-old who enjoys most motor activities. But in group situations, he is easily distracted and has difficulty attending to tasks and waiting. His mother and classroom staff report that Lon often races around, bumping into and falling over objects. At mealtimes, he has difficulty attending to food, stuffs food into his mouth, and often spills a substantial amount on the table and floor.

Aside from food allergies and a severe speech articulation problem, Lon appears to have no other medical concerns. His primary educational handicapping conditions (as determined by the special education team) are delays in speech and language and gross and fine motor development.

Discussion

Lon's test scores must be interpreted and modified with consideration for his young age. Fine motor items requiring skill with pencil and scissor should not be expected of a 3 year-old. Therefore the therapist should not depend solely on the total scores as plotted on the Scoring Profile, but should consider Lon's performance on the gross motor tasks, the pellets in the bottle task, and those aspects of the fine motor tasks related to postural control.

Most of Lon's problems seem to be associated with decreased postural stability/control and processing of primary sensory information (vestibular/proprioceptive/tactile input). Dysfunction in these systems retard development of righting and equilibrium responses, ocular control, skilled movement, motor planning, and the ability to sort out sensory input that allows attention to appropriate information for learning.

As a preschooler, Lon will be participating in an active program with much opportunity for visual and auditory stimulation. It will be critical for him to develop ocular motor control in order to benefit from preschool learning activities. Test scores indicate that Lon's ocular motor control is poor. Before he can improve, however, Lon needs to develop stable neck and head control which will provide the foundation for ocular control and the ability to focus on pertinent stimuli.

Lon is exhibiting attentional difficulties. He requires graded amounts of primary sensory input. Vestibular/proprioceptive/tactile input can have an organizing effect on the central nervous system, providing the inhibition needed to screen out extraneous stimulation and allow for attention to specific information. Lon will need further assessment of oral/motor abilities. Parent and teacher observations seem to indicate that these skills are delayed.

General Therapy Objectives for Lon emphasize improving postural control and movement responses, awareness of body in space, proximal joint control, visual focus and tracking, and attending behavior (starred items). His treatment plan will include activities to enhance sensory development and processing. His program must be carefully structured with the activities graded appropriately. See Individual Treatment Plan for specific examples of appropriate activities.

Sensorimotor Performance Analysis

Name _Lon_
Birthdate
Date of Evaluation _4-26-88_

Age _3_
Evaluator _F. R._
Additional Information

Item A: Rolling

Won't lie down to roll _____ Will not roll _____

		Poor		Optimal
1.	Rolls both directions	1 lt___ rt___	3	(5)
2.	Motor planning	(1) lt___ rt___	3	5
3.	Body righting	1 lt___ rt___	(3)	5
4.	Head righting a. prone b. supine c. lateral	(1) (1) (1)	3 3 3	5 5 5
5.	Asymmetrical tonic neck	1 lt___ rt___	3	(5)
6.	Antigravity flexion	1	(3)	5
7.	Antigravity extension a. hips flexed b. knees flexed c. arms flexed	(1) ✓ ✓	3	5
8.	Becomes dizzy	1	3	(5)

Item B: Belly Crawling

Will not assume or maintain a prone position _____

Will not crawl fast _____

		Poor		Optimal
1.	Motor planning	(1)	3	5
2.	Hand position a. pulls with forearms not hands b. hands fisted c. fingertips only d. palms only e. uses whole hand to pull	1 — — — ✓	3	(5)
3.	Extremity lag	(1) lt ✓ rt UE (LE)	3	5
4.	Propulsion-feet & knees push	1	3	(5)
5.	Antigravity extension	(1)	3	5
6.	Prone head righting	1	(3)	5
7.	Upper trunk extension	1 (2)	3	5
8.	Lateral trunk movement	1	(3)	5
9.	Crawling pattern a. homolateral/ATNR b. homologous/STNR c. reciprocal	1 (2) ✓ ✓	3	5

Notes _Occasionally used homolateral pattern - wouldn't stay prone; kept going into creeping position or would roll over - he was trying to comply and do a good job._

Item C: Bat the Ball from Hands and Knees

		Poor		Optimal
1.	Maintains 4-pt. position	1	3	(5)
2.	Eye tracking	1	(3)	5
3.	Visual avoiding reaction	1	3	(5)
4.	Crosses midline visually	1 lt___ rt___	(3)	5
5.	Crosses midline motorically	(1) lt___ rt___	3	5
6.	Head righting	1	(3)	5
7.	Symmetrical tonic neck	(1)	3	5
8.	Hand position of support arm a. fisted b. fingertips only c. palms only d. whole hand flat	(1) lt ✓ rt ✓ lt___ rt___ lt___ rt___ lt___ rt___	3	5
9.	Hand position of hitting arm a. fisted b. fingertips only c. palms only d. whole hand flat	1 lt___ rt___ lt___ rt___ lt___ rt___ lt___ rt___	3	(5)
10.	Maintains 3-pt. position	(1) lt___ rt___	3	5
11.	Asymmetrical tonic neck	1 lt___ rt___	3	(5)
12.	Shoulder control	1 lt___ rt___	(3)	5
13.	Eye hand coordination	1 lt___ rt___	(3)	5

Item D: Kneeling Balance

Will not assume kneeling position _____

		Poor		Optimal
1.	Assumes kneeling	1	3	(5)
2.	Maintains kneeling position	(1)	3	5
3.	Hip stability	(1)	3	5
4.	Tolerates movement	(1)	3	5
5.	Lateral head righting	(1)	3	5
6.	Trunk righting	(1)	3	5
7.	Extremity righting a. upper extremities b. lower extremities	(1) lt ✓ rt ✓ lt ✓ rt ✓	3	5
8.	Protective extension	(1) lt___ rt___	3	5
9.	Body rotation	(1)	3	5
10.	Antigravity extension	(1)	3	5
11.	Antigravity flexion	(1)	3	5
12.	Symmetrical tonic neck	(1)	3	5
13.	Asymmetrical tonic neck	1 lt___ rt___	3	(5)

Item E: Pellets in Bottle

		Poor		Optimal
1.	Trunk stability	1	3	(5)
2.	Trunk posture	1	3	(5)
3.	Head position	1	3	5
	a. mid-position	lt ✓ rt ___ (1)		
	b. flexed	1	3	(5)
	c. extended	1	3	
4.	Uses unilateral reach	1	3	(5)
5.	Grasp adequate for age	(1)	3	5
	a. palmer grasp			
	b. superior palmer grasp	___		
	c. lateral pinch	___		
	d. inferior pincer grasp	✓		
	e. radial digital grasp			
	f. forefinger pinch			
6.	Mouths or bangs bottle	1	3	(5)
7.	Avoiding reactions	1	3	(5)
8.	Puts pellets in bottle	1	3	(5)
9.	Picks pellets up in sequence	(1)	3	5
10.	Changes hand at mid-line	(1)	3	5
11.	Preferred hand ___	(1)	3	5
12.	Dumps pellets out	1	3	(5)
13.	Tremor	1	3	(5)
14.	Associated reactions	1	3	(5)

Item F: Pencil and Paper Task

		Poor		Optimal
1.	Trunk stability	1	3	(5)
2.	Trunk posture	1	3	(5)
3.	Head position	1	3	(5)
	a. mid-position	lt ___ rt ___		
	b. flexed	1	3 (4)	5
	c. extended	1	3	(5)
4.	Differentiates ends of pencil	1	3	(5)
5.	Positions paper to body center	1	3	(5)
		lt ___ rt ___		
6.	Stabilizes paper with one hand	1	3	(5)
7.	Pencil position	1	(3)	5
	a. gross grasp (fist)	___		
	b. lateral pinch			
	c. radial-digital pinch	✓		
	d. avoids placing fingertips on pencil	___		
	e. thumb/forefinger opposition, pencil resting on 2nd finger	occasionally		
8.	Forearm position	(1)	3	5
9.	Grip strength	1	3 (4)	5
	hypotonic	___		
	hypertonic	___		
10.	Drawing pressure	1	(3 ½)	5
	excessively heavy			
	excessively light	___		
11.	Preferred hand (lt ___ rt ___)	1	3	(5)
	a. switches during testing	1	3	5
	b. draws across body mid-line	(1)	3	
	(twisted body to left)	lt ___ rt ✓		
12.	Imitates strokes	(1)	3	5
	a. vertical			
	b. circular	___		
	c. scribbles	✓		
	d. bangs/mouths pencil			
13.	Copies			
	a. circle	(1)	3	5
	b. cross	(1)	3	5
14.	Upper extremity movement	1	3	(5)
	a. primarily shoulder	___		
	b. elbow/forearm			
	c. wrist/finger	✓		
15.	Associated movements	1	(3)	5
16.	Tremor	1	3	(5)

Item G: Scissor Task

		Poor		Optimal
1.	Trunk stability	1 (2)	3	5
2.	Trunk posture	1	3	(5)
3.	Head position	1	(3)	5
	a. mid-position	lt ___ rt ✓		
	b. flexed	1	3	(5)
	c. extended	1	3	(5)
4.	Shoulder position	(1)	3	5
5.	Forearm holding paper	(1)	3	5
	a. pronated	✓		
	b. supinated			
6.	Hand grip holding paper	1	(3)	5
	a. hypotonic	✓		
	b. hypertonic	___		
7.	Forearm cutting paper	(1)	3	5
	a. pronated	✓		
	b. supinated			
8.	Wrist position during cutting	(1)	3	5
	a. flexion	✓		
	b. extension	___		
	c. ulnar deviation	___		
9.	Hand cutting paper	(1)	3	5
	a. lateral pinch	✓		
	b. forefinger pinch			
	c. thumb/hand opposition	___		
10.	Unused fingers-cutting hand	(1)	3	5
11.	Visual orienting	1	3	(5)
12.	Cut is continuous/smooth	(1)	3	5
13.	Straight line is accurate	(1)	3	5
14.	Curved line is accurate	(1)	3	5
15.	Preferred hand lt ___ rt ✓	1	3	(5)
16.	Tremor	1	3	(5)
17.	Associated reactions	(1)	3	5

Reflex Activity Assessment

	REFLEX OR RESPONSE	Poor-Optimal		
Spinal	TACTILE DEFENSIVENESS	P	(F)	A
BRAIN STEM	ASYMMETRICAL TONIC NECK-RIGHT	P	F	A
	AYMMETRICAL TONIC NECK-LEFT	P	F	A
	SYMMETRICAL TONIC NECK	(P)	F	A
	ANTIGRAVITY FLEXION	P	(✓) F	A
	ANTIGRAVITY EXTENSION	P	F	A
	ASSOCIATED REACTIONS	P	F	A
MID BRAIN	NECK RIGHTING	P	(F)	A
	BODY RIGHTING	A	F (✓)	P
	HEAD RIGHTING-PRONE	A	F (✓)	P
	HEAD RIGHTING-SUPINE	A	F	(P)
AUTO-MATIC	STARTLE	P	F	A
	LANDAU	P	F	A
	PROTECTIVE EXTENSION	A	F	(P)

CORTICAL	EQUILIBRIUM REACTIONS	RT.	LT.
	PRONE — HEAD RTG.	A (F) P	A (F) P
	SUPINE — TRUNK RTG.	A F (✓)P	A (F) P
	(SITTING) — PROTECTIVE EXT.	A (F)P	A (F) P
	KNEELING — EXTREMITIES	A (F) P	A (F) P

Notes *Used small tilt board, he was inconsistent on these responses; sometimes slow to respond or would get response initially but lose it and fall.*

slight

Eye Tracking: (Midline jerk) isolated eye movement poor, visual avoidance, nystagmus

Vertical: *would follow upward, not downward*

Horizontal: *when cross midline - stops*

Convergence: *No*

Thumb-Finger Circles: Sequence, speed, fingertips, accuracy, reverse-pattern, mirroring, intent concentration

Could not do
no sequence or accuracy, poor planning *No*

Rapid Hand Movement: (Speed) accuracy of placement, tone, sequence, asymmetry

usually only moved right hand
occasionally alternated - hands were floppy, speed very slow

Localization of Tactile Stimuli: Estimate distances off

Would get some correct, usually would choose the finger next to the correct one and then the correct one.

Muscle Tone: Increased, decreased, fluctuating

Slight Low tone

Distribution: neck/trunk, (UE, LE, oral/facial) asymmetrical

Oral Motor Function: Hyper-sensitivity, oral self-stimulation, feeding problems

Sensory Behaviors: Vestibular, proprioceptive, tactile, visual, auditory, gustatory

Precautions:

Sensorimotor Performance Analysis
Scoring Profile

Category	Total Score	Maximum Score
ATNR	28	35
STNR	7	15
Anti-gravity Extension	48	70
Anti-gravity Flexion	20	30
Body righting/Trunk flexibility	21	40
Head righting	18	35
Equilibrium/Protective reactions	23	50
Vestibular Function	31	75
Tactile Processing	29	40
Visual Processing	44	70
Bilateral Integration	64	115
Motor Planning	61	125
Tone & Strength	80	110
Stability/Mobility	91	170
Neuro Status	52	80
Developmental Level	79	140

Test columns: A – Rolling, B – Belly Crawling, C – Bat the Ball, D – Kneel Standing, E – Pellets, F – Pencil & Paper, G – Scissors

Name _____ Age 3

Evaluator LOM ER _____ Case Manager _____

Date 4-26-88

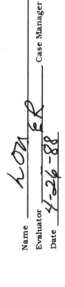

Occupational/Physical Therapy Department
General Therapy Objectives

Name: _Lon_____   Therapist(s): _____F.R._____

Schedule: _____   Date: _01/15/88_____

Sensory-Related Goals

	_____	Decrease oversensitivity to sensory stimulation
	_____	Decrease tactile defensiveness
*	_X_	Develop awareness of body in space
	_____	Increase activity level
	_X_	Decrease activity level
	_____	Decrease self-stimulating activities

Gross Motor Goals

*	_X_	Improve postural control and movement responses (balance)
	_X_	Improve developmental skills
	_____	Increase strength
	_____	Increase flexibility
	_____	Increase endurance
*	_X_	Improve gross motor planning (ability to plan and carry out coordinated movement)

Fine Motor Goals

*	_X_	Improve shoulder control
	_____	Develop gross grasp and release
	_____	Improve hand/finger coordination and manipulation skills
	_____	Improve bilateral coordination
	_X_	Improve fine motor planning skills
	_____	Improve daily living skills

Visual Goals

*	_X_	Improve visual focus and attention
	_X_	Improve eye tracking skills
	_X_	Improve eye/hand coordination

Behavioral Goals

*	_X_	Improve attending behaviors
	_X_	Increase group interaction
	_X_	Improve ability to follow directions

Occupational/Physical Therapy
Individual Treatment Plan

Name: _Lon_

Age: _3_   Rm: _102_

Teacher: _Mrs. Smith_

Precautions: _____

Therapist: _F.R._   Date: _01/15/88_

Major Objectives

1. *Improve postural control for functional play activities.*
2. *Improve attending skills.*
3. *Increase awareness of body space.*

Specific Objectives

1 a. Lon will maintain a kneeling position while engaged in a simple fine motor task for 5 minutes.

b. Lon will squat and return to standing while transferring toys from the floor to the table, 2 of 3 trials.

2. Lon will play on task for 5 minutes without getting up to run away.

3 Lon will move himself from his classroom to the therapy room without bumping the walls or falling down.

Treatment Plan

CNS Preparation: *Decrease visual input; grade slow vestibular and proprioceptive input to increase tone and proximal stability.*

- *Swing gently (head to toe direction) clinging to bolster swing*
- *Prone in hammock or innertube, child propels self by pushing off the ground or grasping therapist's hand and pulling*
- *Magic carpet — child pulls a classmate down a carpeted hall on a piece of heavy plastic or, if the hall flooring is linoleum, on a rug*

Sensory Activities: *Tactile, deep pressure*

- *Pretend to wash body parts with a washcloth*
- *Child rubs lotion all over face, arms, legs, feet and tummy*
- *Roll in carpeted barrel*

Oral and Pre-speech Activities: *Needs a functional feeding evaluation; provide heavy pressure to face and around mouth with puppet play, hugs and kisses; brush teeth with an electric toothbrush.*

Gross Motor Activities:

•*Roll up/down incline; arms overhead/down at sides; supine hug/squeeze pillows with arms and legs, etc.*

Fine Motor-Manipulative Activities:

• *Squeeze toys, waterplay (gross grasp), Play-doh*
• *From supine, bat suspended ball, swing scarves*

Visual Skills:

• *Flashlight tag on the ceiling (from supine); flashlight tracking games*
• *Marble tracking toys*
• *From supine, visually follow and hit at suspended objects (balls, balloons, etc.)*

Behavior:

• *Keep activities short and structured, minimize visual distractions*
• *Treat in very small group or one-to-one*
• *Keep directions short and simple*

A Child with Mild Retardation

Vera is an overweight 8 year-old who wears glasses for myopia. Extremely distractable and impulsive, Vera has a low frustration tolerance and, when presented with difficult or unfamiliar tasks, will engage in manipulative behaviors to avoid the task. She needs constant encouragement, structure, and redirection to complete a task. Vera interacts little with peers, frequently seeking attention from adults. She is a student at a special school for mentally retarded children aged five through 21. There are 21 other children in her class, but the class is one of several classes in one area in an open school.

Discussion

Although Vera is a fairly high-functioning child cognitively, test scores indicate that she has significant sensorimotor problems. It is important that she be able to function in group situations and interact with her peers. Tactile processing problems appear to be contributing to her difficulties in these areas. Lack of appropriate pain response is also a concern. Vera's insecurity in space is preventing her from engaging in normal childhood motor activities. Limitation of motor activity results in less exposure to primary sensory stimulation needed to develop good postural control, muscle tone, and movement responses. Limited motor activity is also probably contributing to her overweight condition and poor endurance.

Vera's treatment program will have to provide intensive tactile, vestibular, and proprioceptive input, graded as she can tolerate (see *Individual Treatment Plan* for specific suggestions). Activities will be chosen which emphasize input to the tactile/vestibular/proprioceptive systems while facilitating body righting, head righting, improved postural responses, and simple motor planning.

Sensorimotor Performance Analysis

Name ___Vera___   Age ___8___

Birthdate _____   Evaluator ___R.S.___

Date of Evaluation _____   Additional Information _____

Item A: Rolling

Won't lie down to roll_____Will not roll _____

		Poor		Optimal
1.	Rolls both directions	1 lt___ rt___	3	(5)
2.	Motor planning	1 lt___ rt**2**	3	5
3.	Body righting	1 lt___ rt**2**	3	5
4.	Head righting a. prone b. supine c. lateral	1 1 1	3 (3) (3)	(5) 5 5
5.	Asymmetrical tonic neck	1 lt___ rt___	3	(5)
6.	Antigravity flexion	1	3	(5)
7.	Antigravity extension a. hips flexed b. knees flexed c. arms flexed	(1) ✓ ✓ ✓	3	5
8.	Becomes dizzy	1	3	(5)

Item B: Belly Crawling

Will not assume or maintain a prone position _____

Will not crawl fast _____

		Poor		Optimal
1.	Motor planning	1	3	(5)
2.	Hand position a. pulls with forearms not hands b. hands fisted c. fingertips only d. palms only e. uses whole hand to pull	(1) ✓ ___ ___ ___ ___	3	5
3.	Extremity lag	1 lt___ rt___ UE/LE	3	(5)
4.	Propulsion-feet & knees push	1	3	(5)
5.	Antigravity extension	1	(3)	5
6.	Prone head righting	1	(3)	5
7.	Upper trunk extension	1 (2)	3	5
8.	Lateral trunk movement	1	(3)	5
9.	Crawling pattern a. homolateral/ATNR b. homologous/STNR c. reciprocal	1 ✓ ___	(3)	5 ✓

Notes _Tires quickly_
Item D.- very insecure and
fearful; holds on to tiltboard
at slightest tilt.

Item C: Bat the Ball from Hands and Knees

		Poor		Optimal
1.	Maintains 4-pt. position	1	3	(5)
2.	Eye tracking	1	(3)	5
3.	Visual avoiding reaction	(1)	3	5
4.	Crosses midline visually	1 lt___ rt___	(3)	5
5.	Crosses midline motorically	1 lt___ rt___	(3)	5
6.	Head righting	1	(3)	5
7.	Symmetrical tonic neck	1	(3)	5
8.	Hand position of support arm a. fisted b. fingertips only c. palms only d. whole hand flat	1 (2) 3 lt___ rt___ lt✓ rt✓ lt___ rt___ lt___ rt___		5
9.	Hand position of hitting arm a. fisted b. fingertips only c. palms only d. whole hand flat	1 (2) 3 lt___ rt___ lt___ rt___ lt✓ rt✓ lt___ rt___		5
10.	Maintains 3-pt. position	1 lt___ rt___	(3)	5
11.	Asymmetrical tonic neck	1 lt___ rt___	3	(5)
12.	Shoulder control	1 lt___ rt___	3 (4)	5
13.	Eye hand coordination	1 lt___ rt___	(3)	5

Item D: Kneeling Balance

Will not assume kneeling position_____

		Poor		Optimal
1.	Assumes kneeling	1	3 (4)	5
2.	Maintains kneeling position	1	(3)	5
3.	Hip stability	1	(3)	5
4.	Tolerates movement	1 (2)	3	5
5.	Lateral head righting	1	3 (4)	5
6.	Trunk righting	1	(3)	5
7.	Extremity righting a. upper extremities b. lower extremities	1 lt___ rt___ lt___ rt___	(3)	5
8.	Protective extension	1 lt___ rt___	(3)	5
9.	Body rotation	1	(3)	5
10.	Antigravity extension	1	(3)	5
11.	Antigravity flexion	1	3	(5)
12.	Symmetrical tonic neck	1	3	(5)
13.	Asymmetrical tonic neck	1 lt___ rt___	3	(5)

Item E: Pellets in Bottle

		Poor		Optimal
1.	Trunk stability	1	3	(5)
2.	Trunk posture	1	(3)	5
3.	Head position	1	3	(5)
	a. mid-position	lt__ rt__		
	b. flexed	1	3 (4)	5
	c. extended	1	3	(5)
4.	Uses unilateral reach	1	3	(5)
5.	Grasp adequate for age	(1)	3	5
	a. palmer grasp			
	b. superior palmer grasp	___		
	c. lateral pinch	___		
	d. inferior pincer grasp	✓		
	e. radial digital grasp	✓		
	f. forefinger pinch			
6.	Mouths or bangs bottle	1	3	(5)
7.	Avoiding reactions	1	(3)	5
8.	Puts pellets in bottle	1	3	(5)
9.	Picks pellets up in sequence	1	3	(5)
10.	Changes hand at mid-line	1	3	(5)
11.	Preferred hand ____	1	3	(5)
12.	Dumps pellets out	1	3	(5)
13.	Tremor	1	3	(5)
14.	Associated reactions	1	(3)	5

Item F: Pencil and Paper Task

		Poor		Optimal
1.	Trunk stability	1	3	(5)
2.	Trunk posture	1	(3)	5
3.	Head position	1	3	(5)
	a. mid-position	lt__ rt__		
	b. flexed	1	3 (4)	5
	c. extended	1	3	(5)
4.	Differentiates ends of pencil	1	3	(5)
5.	Positions paper to body center	1	3	(5)
		lt__ rt__		
6.	Stabilizes paper with one hand	1	3	(5)
7.	Pencil position	(1)	3	5
	a. gross grasp (fist)			
	b. lateral pinch	✓		
	c. radial-digital pinch	___		
	d. avoids placing fingertips on pencil	✓		
	e. thumb/forefinger opposition, pencil resting on 2nd finger			
8.	Forearm position	1	3	(5)
9.	Grip strength	1	3 (4)	5
	hypotonic	___		
	hypertonic			
10.	Drawing pressure	1	3 (4)	5
	excessively heavy			
	excessively light	✓		
11.	Preferred hand (lt__ rt__)			
	a. switches during testing	1	3	(5)
	b. draws across body mid-line	1	3	(5)
		lt__ rt ✓		
12.	Imitates strokes	1	3	(5)
	a. vertical	✓		
	b. circular	✓		
	c. scribbles			
	d. bangs/mouths pencil	___		
13.	Copies			
	a. circle	1	3	(5)
	b. cross	1	3	(5)
14.	Upper extremity movement	1	3	(5)
	a. primarily shoulder	___		
	b. elbow/forearm	___		
	c. wrist/finger			
15.	Associated movements	1	(3)	5
16.	Tremor	1	3	(5)

Item G: Scissor Task

		Poor		Optimal
1.	Trunk stability	1	3	(5)
2.	Trunk posture	1	(3)	5
3.	Head position	1	3	(5)
	a. mid-position	lt__ rt__		
	b. flexed	1	3 (4)	5
	c. extended	1	3	(5)
4.	Shoulder position	1	3 (4)	5
5.	Forearm holding paper	1	3	(5)
	a. pronated			
	b. supinated	___		
6.	Hand grip holding paper	1	3	(5)
	a. hypotonic			
	b. hypertonic	___		
7.	Forearm cutting paper	1	3	(5)
	a. pronated			
	b. supinated	___		
8.	Wrist position during cutting	1	3 (4)	5
	a. flexion	✓		
	b. extension	___		
	c. ulnar deviation	___		
9.	Hand cutting paper	(1)	3	5
	a. lateral pinch	✓		
	b. forefinger pinch			
	c. thumb/hand opposition	___		
10.	Unused fingers-cutting hand	1	(3)	5
11.	Visual orienting	1	3 (4)	5
12.	Cut is continuous/smooth	1	(3)	5 *choppy*
13.	Straight line is accurate	1	3 (4)	5
14.	Curved line is accurate	1	(3)	5
15.	Preferred hand	1	3	(5)
	lt__ rt__			
16.	Tremor	1	3	(5)
17.	Associated reactions	1	(3)	5

Reflex Activity Assessment

REFLEX OR RESPONSE — Poor-Optimal

Spinal	TACTILE DEFENSIVENESS	P	(F✓)	A
BRAIN STEM	ASYMMETRICAL TONIC NECK-RIGHT	P	(F)	A
	AYMMETRICAL TONIC NECK-LEFT	P	(F)	A
	SYMMETRICAL TONIC NECK	P	F ✓	A
	ANTIGRAVITY FLEXION	P	(F)	A
	ANTIGRAVITY EXTENSION	P	F	(A)
	ASSOCIATED REACTIONS	P	(F)	A
MID BRAIN	NECK RIGHTING	P	F	(A)
	BODY RIGHTING	A	(F)	P
	HEAD RIGHTING-PRONE	A	(F)	P
	HEAD RIGHTING-SUPINE	A	(F)	P
AUTO-MATIC	STARTLE	P	F	(A)
	LANDAU	P	F	(A)
	PROTECTIVE EXTENSION	A	(F)	P

	EQUILIBRIUM REACTIONS		RT.			LT.	
COR-TICAL	PRONE — HEAD RTG.	A	(F)	P	(A)	F	P
	SUPINE — TRUNK RTG.	A	(F)	P	(A)	F	P
	SITTING — PROTECTIVE EXT.	A	(F)	P	A	(F)	P
	KNEELING — EXTREMITIES	A	(F)	P	A	(F)	P

Notes ___ tiltboard used ___

Eye Tracking: (Midline jerk) isolated eye movement poor, visual avoidance, nystagmus

Vertical: *Difficulty following without moving head*

Horizontal:

Convergence: *No convergence*

Thumb-Finger Circles: Sequence, speed, fingertips, accuracy, reverse-pattern, mirroring, intent concentration

Unable to isolate fingertips
Unable to sequence
Associated movements pronounced

Rapid Hand Movement: (Speed) (accuracy of placement) (tone,) sequence, asymmetry

Vera unable to do with any speed, double clapping much of time,
Very floppy - poor tone
Had difficulty supinating

Localization of Tactile Stimuli: Estimate distances off

Was able to localize fairly well, but was extremely uncomfortable
during this portion of test. Mom states Vera has decreased
Pain sensation.

Muscle Tone: Increased, (decreased) fluctuating
overall

Distribution: neck/trunk, UE, LE, oral/facial, asymmetrical

Oral Motor Function: (Hyper-sensitivity) (oral self-stimulation,) feeding problems

Doesn't like people touching face
Sucks on objects, toys, clothing, etc.

Sensory Behaviors: (Vestibular) (proprioceptive,) (tactile,) (visual,) auditory, gustatory

Perseverative
Poor tone, stability, poor body awareness,
teacher talks of difficulty in groups.

Precautions:

Seizure disorder

Sensorimotor Performance Analysis
Scoring Profile

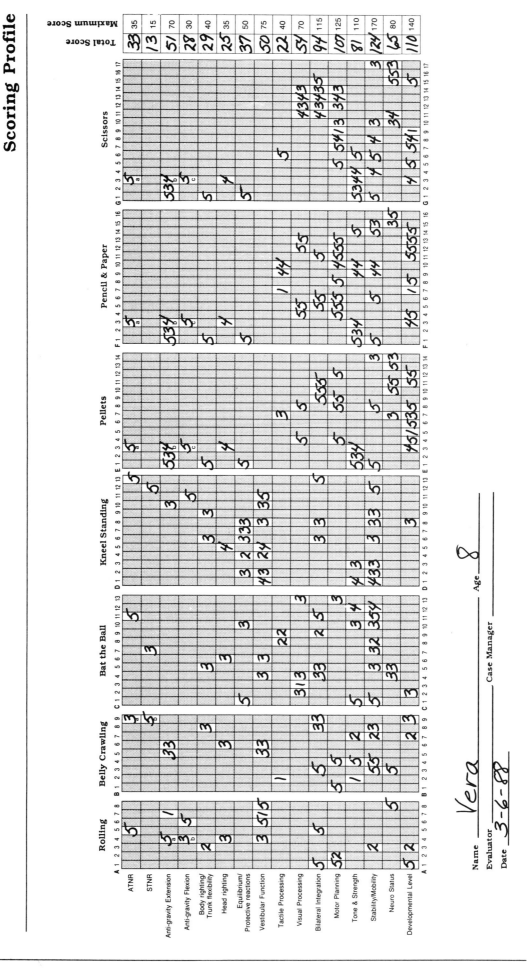

Name __Vera__ Age __8__

Evaluator _____ Case Manager _____

Date __3-6-88__

Occupational/Physical Therapy Department
General Therapy Objectives

Name: _Vera_   Therapist(s): _R.S._

Schedule: _____   Date: _01/15/88_

Sensory-Related Goals
*   _X_   Decrease oversensitivity to sensory stimulation
*   _X_   Decrease tactile defensiveness
*   _X_   Develop awareness of body in space
      _X_   Increase activity level
      _____ Decrease activity level
      _____ Decrease self-stimulating activities

Gross Motor Goals
*   _X_   Improve postural control and movement responses (balance)
      _X_   Improve developmental skills
      _X_   Increase strength
      _____ Increase flexibility
*   _X_   Increase endurance
      _X_   Improve gross motor planning (ability to plan and carry out coordinated movement)

Fine Motor Goals
*   _X_   Improve shoulder control
      _X_   Develop gross grasp and release
      _X_   Improve hand/finger coordination and manipulation skills
      _____ Improve bilateral coordination
      _X_   Improve fine motor planning skills
      _____ Improve daily living skills

Visual Goals
*   _X_   Improve visual focus and attention
      _X_   Improve eye tracking skills
      _X_   Improve eye/hand coordination

Behavioral Goals
*   _X_   Improve attending behaviors
      _X_   Increase group interaction
      _____ Improve ability to follow directions

Occupational/Physical Therapy
Individual Treatment Plan

Name: _Vera_

Age: _8_   Rm: _104_

Teacher: _Mrs. Green_

Precautions: _____

Therapist: _R.S._   Date: _01/15/88_

Major Objectives

1. Decrease tactile defensiveness and increase tactile discrimination
2. Improve tolerance of movement activities for motor planning
3. Improve postural control and movement responses (balance and righting reactions)
4. Increase endurance during motor activities

Specific Objectives

1a. Vera will tolerate therapist touching her without pulling away. and without facial grimaces, 100 percent of the time.
  b. She will tolerate input from a variety of textures without grimacing or pulling away, 2 of 3 trials.
2a. Vera will climb onto trampoline and bounce (either sitting or supine) independently and without fearfulness, 100 percent of the time.
  b. Vera will attempt activities on unstable surfaces without fear twice during a 10 minute free play session.
3. Vera will demonstrate consistent segmentation of hips and shoulders, as well as supine and lateral head righting responses during rolling.
4. Vera will be able to perform 2 gross motor tasks without becoming fatigued (i.e., sighing, lying down on floor, etc.).

Treatment Plan

CNS Preparation: _Excitatory_
• _Vigorous swinging in hammock; short revolutions_
• _Bounce on trampoline in sitting position_

Sensory Activities:
• _Tactile -- rub arms, legs, face with washcloth and/or lotion; rub/squirm on carpet._
• _Vestibular (see CNS Preparation)._

Oral and Pre-Speech Activities: _Tactile activities to facial area — carefully graded (see sensory activities)._

Gross Motor Activities:

- *Belly crawl on smooth surface and then on carpet all directions*
- *Scooter board (in prone) through an obstacle course; down a ramp*
- *In prone, rock onto right side and then onto left with arms over head*

Fine Motor-Manipulative Activities:

- *While prone, hang onto a hoop while being pulled on the scooter board*
- *Search for objects hidden in sand*
- *Place pegs (of various sizes) in peg board*
- *Slip clothes pins onto the lip of a coffee can*

Visual Skills:

- *Flashlight tracking games in the dark*
- *Trace a trail on the blackboard using a flashlight*
- *Bat at suspended equipment from supine*

Behavior:

- *Have Vera repeat directions; keep instructions simple and activities structured.*
- *Provide opportunities for her to help instruct other children.*

A Teenager With
Motor and Mental Handicaps

Cindy is a 19 year-old whose development was normal until she was 9 years old. At that time, she was admitted to the hospital for an emergency appendectomy. She arrested during surgery and was comatose for the next two years. After she came out of the coma, it was apparent that Cindy had sustained neurological damage. Subsequent treatment and testing indicate her condition is improving slowly.

Cindy exhibits hypertonicity in all four extremities, the left side being more severe than the right. No limitation of range of motion is noted. Cindy can follow directions, but is easily distracted and excited by auditory and visual stimuli (such as lights). When excited, she giggles, her speech becomes louder and breathier, and her rigidity increases. Gross motor activities are limited because of her lack of normal balance reactions. Cindy's movements are stiff, and she lacks control of movement in the midranges, i.e. she collapses into her wheelchair rather than lowering herself into it.

When moving in and out of various positions, Cindy has difficulty breaking up total patterns.

Discussion

Cindy is dominated by flexor patterns in all positions. She also demonstrates strong primitive reflex responses. Hypersensitive to auditory and visual stimulation, she frequently exhibits increased rigidity with attempted voluntary movement.

A treatment program for Cindy will emphasize normalization of muscle tone; development of righting and equilibrium responses (including extension patterns and body rotation); and decreased hypersensitivity to sensory stimulation. Treatment should also provide adequate input for improved awareness of body in space and attending behaviors. Cindy needs improved bilateral coordination for developing fine motor skills, etc.

Sensorimotor Performance Analysis

Name ___Cindy___ Age ___16___

Birthdate _____ Evaluator _____

Date of Evaluation ___2-17-88___ Additional Information _____

Item A: Rolling

Won't lie down to roll _____ Will not roll _____

	Poor		Optimal
1. Rolls both directions lt___ rt___	1	3	(5)
2. Motor planning lt___ rt___	(1)	3	5
3. Body righting lt___ rt___	(1)	3	5
4. Head righting a. prone b. supine c. lateral	(1) (1) (1)	3 3 3	5 5 5
5. Asymmetrical tonic neck lt___ rt___	1	3	(5)
6. Antigravity flexion	1	3	(5)
7. Antigravity extension a. hips flexed b. knees flexed c. arms flexed	(1) ___ ___	3	5
8. Becomes dizzy	1	(3)	5

Item B: Belly Crawling

Will not assume or maintain a prone position _Maintains prone or prone on elbows for maximum 15 seconds_

Will not crawl fast _____

Cannot belly crawl

	Poor		Optimal
1. Motor planning	O 1	3	5
2. Hand position a. pulls with forearms not hands b. hands fisted c. fingertips only d. palms only e. uses whole hand to pull	O 1 ___ ___ ___ ___	3	5
3. Extremity lag lt___ rt___ UE/LE	O 1	3	5
4. Propulsion-feet & knees push	O 1	3	5
5. Antigravity extension	O 1	3	5
6. Prone head righting	O 1	3	5
7. Upper trunk extension	O 1	3	5
8. Lateral trunk movement	O 1	3	5
9. Crawling pattern a. homolateral/ATNR b. homologous/STNR c. reciprocal	O 1 ___ ___ ___	3	5

Item C: Bat the Ball from Hands and Knees

	Poor		Optimal
1. Maintains 4-pt. position	1	(3) _momentarily_	5
2. Eye tracking	1	(3)	5
3. Visual avoiding reaction	1	3	(5)
4. Crosses midline visually lt___ rt___	(1)	3	5
5. Crosses midline motorically lt___ rt___	(1)	3	5
6. Head righting	1	3	(5)
7. Symmetrical tonic neck	(1)	3	5
8. Hand position of support arm a. fisted lt✔ rt✔ b. fingertips only lt___ rt___ c. palms only lt___ rt___ d. whole hand flat lt___ rt___	(1)	3	5
9. Hand position of hitting arm a. fisted lt✔ rt✔ b. fingertips only lt___ rt___ c. palms only lt___ rt___ d. whole hand flat lt___ rt___	(1)	3	5
10. Maintains 3-pt. position lt___ rt___	(1)	3	5
11. Asymmetrical tonic neck lt___ rt___	(1)	3	5
12. Shoulder control lt___ rt___	(1)	3	5
13. Eye hand coordination lt___ rt___	(1)	3	5

Item D: Kneeling Balance

Will not assume kneeling position _____

	Poor		Optimal
1. Assumes kneeling	1	(3)	5
2. Maintains kneeling position	O 1	3	5
3. Hip stability	O 1	3	5
4. Tolerates movement	O 1	3	5
5. Lateral head righting	O 1	3	5
6. Trunk righting	O 1	3	5
7. Extremity righting a. upper extremities lt___ rt___ b. lower extremities lt___ rt___	O 1	3	5
8. Protective extension lt___ rt___	O 1	3	5
9. Body rotation	O 1	3	5
10. Antigravity extension	O 1	3	5
11. Antigravity flexion	O 1	3	5
12. Symmetrical tonic neck	O 1	3	5
13. Asymmetrical tonic neck lt___ rt___	O 1	3	5

Notes _Item C - Can get up on all fours position - can't lift one arm up for 3-pt. When asked to bat ball she sits back on heels. Item D. - To maintain kneeling position Cindy must hold on or lean on something - hips always flexed._

Item E: Pellets in Bottle

	Poor		Optimal
1. Trunk stability	①	3	5
2. Trunk posture	①	3	5
3. Head position	①	3	5
a. mid-position lt ✓ rt___			
b. flexed	①	3	5
c. extended	1	3	⑤
4. Uses unilateral reach	1	3	⑤
5. Grasp adequate for age	①	3	5
a. palmer grasp ✓			
b. superior palmer grasp			
c. lateral pinch			
d. inferior pincer grasp			
e. radial digital grasp			
f. forefinger pinch			
6. Mouths or bangs bottle	1	3	⑤
7. Avoiding reactions	1	3	⑤
8. Puts pellets in bottle	1	③	5
9. Picks pellets up in sequence	①	3	5
10. Changes hand at mid-line	①	3	5
11. Preferred hand ___	①	3	5
12. Dumps pellets out	1	3	⑤
13. Tremor	1	3	⑤
14. Associated reactions	①	3	5

Item F: Pencil and Paper Task

	Poor		Optimal
1. Trunk stability	①	3	5
2. Trunk posture	①	3	5
3. Head position	①	3	5
a. mid-position lt___ rt X			
b. flexed	①	3	5
c. extended	1	3	⑤
4. Differentiates ends of pencil	1	3	⑤
5. Positions paper to body center	①	3	5
lt ✓ rt___			
6. Stabilizes paper with one hand	1	3	⑤
7. Pencil position	①	3	5
a. gross grasp (fist) ✓			
b. lateral pinch			
c. radial-digital pinch			
d. avoids placing fingertips on pencil			
e. thumb/forefinger opposition, pencil resting on 2nd finger			
8. Forearm position	①	3	5
9. Grip strength	①	3	5
hypotonic			
hypertonic ✓			
10. Drawing pressure	1	3	⑤
excessively heavy			
excessively light			
11. Preferred hand (lt___ rt ✓)			
a. switches during testing	1	3	⑤
b. draws across body mid-line	①	3	5
lt___ rt___			
12. Imitates strokes	①	3	5
a. vertical			
b. circular			
c. scribbles ✓			
d. bangs/mouths pencil			
13. Copies			
a. circle	①	3	5
b. cross	①	3	5
14. Upper extremity movement	①	3	5
a. primarily shoulder ✓			
b. elbow/forearm			
c. wrist/finger			
15. Associated movements	①	3	5
16. Tremor	1	3	⑤

Item G: Scissor Task

	Poor		Optimal
1. Trunk stability	0 1	3	5
2. Trunk posture	0 1	3	5
3. Head position	①	3	5
a. mid-position lt ✓ rt___			
b. flexed	①	3	5
c. extended	1	3	⑤
4. Shoulder position	0 1	3	5
5. Forearm holding paper	0 1	3	5
a. pronated			
b. supinated			
6. Hand grip holding paper	0 1	3	5
a. hypotonic			
b. hypertonic			
7. Forearm cutting paper	0 1	3	5
a. pronated			
b. supinated			
8. Wrist position during cutting	0 1	3	5
a. flexion			
b. extension			
c. ulnar deviation			
9. Hand cutting paper	0 1	3	5
a. lateral pinch			
b. forefinger pinch			
c. thumb/hand opposition			
10. Unused fingers-cutting hand	0 1	3	5
11. Visual orienting	0 1	3	5
12. Cut is continuous/smooth	0 1	3	5
13. Straight line is accurate	0 1	3	5
14. Curved line is accurate	0 1	3	5
15. Preferred hand lt___ rt___	0 1	3	5
16. Tremor	0 1	3	5
17. Associated reactions	0 1	3	5

Reflex Activity Assessment

	REFLEX OR RESPONSE	Poor	—	Optimal
Spinal	TACTILE DEFENSIVENESS	P	F	Ⓐ
BRAIN STEM	ASYMMETRICAL TONIC NECK-RIGHT	Ⓟ	F	A
	AYMMETRICAL TONIC NECK-LEFT	Ⓟ	F	A
	SYMMETRICAL TONIC NECK	Ⓟ	F	A
	ANTIGRAVITY FLEXION	P	F	Ⓐ
	ANTIGRAVITY EXTENSION	Ⓟ	F	A
	ASSOCIATED REACTIONS	Ⓟ	F	A
MID BRAIN	NECK RIGHTING	Ⓟ	F	A
	BODY RIGHTING	Ⓐ	F	P
	HEAD RIGHTING-PRONE	A	F	Ⓟ
	HEAD RIGHTING-SUPINE	A	F	Ⓟ
AUTOMATIC	STARTLE	P	F	A
	LANDAU	P	F	A
	PROTECTIVE EXTENSION	A	Ⓕ	P

	EQUILIBRIUM REACTIONS	RT.			LT.		
COR-TICAL	PRONE HEAD RTG.	Ⓐ	F	P	Ⓐ	F	P
	SUPINE TRUNK RTG.	Ⓐ	F	P	Ⓐ	F	P
	SITTING PROTECTIVE EXT.	A	Ⓕ	P	Ⓐ	F	P
	KNEELING EXTREMITIES	Ⓐ	F	P	A	Ⓕ	P

Notes _Item 6 - Attempted but could not do._

Also - positive supporting reactions

Eye Tracking: Midline jerk, isolated eye movement poor, visual avoidance, nystagmus

Vertical: *Cannot cross mid-line*

Horizontal: *distracted - follows*

Convergence: *Some*

Thumb-Finger Circles: Sequence, speed, fingertips, accuracy, reverse-pattern, mirroring, intent concentration

Unable to do - Could not sequence, could not isolate movements

Rapid Hand Movement: Speed, accuracy of placement, tone, sequence, asymmetry

Unable to do

Localization of Tactile Stimuli: Estimate distances off

Cindy has poor awareness of body + spatial + directional concepts - this was not tested.

Muscle Tone: (Increased) decreased, fluctuating

All four extremities

Distribution: neck/trunk, UE, LE, oral/facial, asymmetrical

When she talks or laughs, tone goes up

Oral Motor Function: Hyper-sensitivity, oral self-stimulation, feeding problems

No feeding problems

Sensory Behaviors: Vestibular, proprioceptive, tactile, visual, auditory, gustatory

Overly sensitive to visual and auditory stimuli -- pupils dilated most of time.

Precautions:

Sensorimotor Performance Analysis
Scoring Profile

	Total Score	Maximum Score
ATNR	9	35
STNR	1	15
Anti-gravity Extension	9	70
Anti-gravity Flexion	21	30
Body righting/Trunk flexibility	4	40
Head righting	9	35
Equilibrium/Protective reactions	6	50
Vestibular Function	19	75
Tactile Processing	14	40
Visual Processing	26	70
Bilateral Integration	24	115
Motor Planning	41	125
Tone & Strength	22	110
Stability/Mobility	32	170
Neuro Status	24	80
Developmental Level	48	140

Columns (left to right): Rolling — Belly Crawling — Bat the Ball — Kneel Standing — Pellets — Pencil & Paper — Scissors

Name Cindy

Evaluator ERJ

Date 2-17-88

Age 16

Case Manager

Occupational/Physical Therapy Department
General Therapy Objectives

Name: _Cindy_____   Therapist(s): _J.G._____

Schedule: _____   Date: _01/15/88_____

Sensory-Related Goals
*   __X___   Decrease oversensitivity to sensory stimulation
   _____   Decrease tactile defensiveness
   *_X___   Develop awareness of body in space
   _____   Increase activity level
   _____   Decrease activity level
   _____   Decrease self-stimulating activities

Gross Motor Goals
*   __X___   Improve postural control and movement responses (balance)
   __X___   Improve developmental skills
   _____   Increase strength
*   __X___   Increase flexibility
   _____   Increase endurance
*   __X___   Improve gross motor planning (ability to plan and carry out coordinated movement)

Fine Motor Goals
   _____   Improve shoulder control
   __X___   Develop gross grasp and release
   __X___   Improve hand/finger coordination and manipulation skills
*   __X___   Improve bilateral coordination
*   __X___   Improve fine motor planning skills
   _____   Improve daily living skills

Visual Goals
*   __X___   Improve visual focus and attention
   __X___   Improve eye tracking skills
   __X___   Improve eye/hand coordination

Behavioral Goals
*   __X___   Improve attending behaviors
   _____   Increase group interaction
   __X___   Improve ability to follow directions

Occupational/Physical Therapy
Individual Treatment Plan

Name: _Cindy_

Age: _19_   Rm: _303_

Teacher: _Mrs. Black_

Precautions: _____

Therapist: _J.G._   Date: _01/15/88_

Major Objectives

1. *Decrease oversensitivity to sensory stimulation*
2. *Normalize muscle tone for increased flexibility, body rotation, and graded motor control.*
3. *Improve equilibrium and protective responses in all positions*
4. *Improve bilateral integration and motor planning skills.*

Specific Objectives

1. *Cindy will be able to participate in therapy session with the lights on without exhibiting increased rigidity.*
2. *Standing facing her wheelchair, Cindy will turn and sit without collapsing into the chair, 100 percent of the time.*
3. *Cindy will use protective responses when tipped laterally off balance from a sitting position, 2 of 3 trials.*
4. *Cindy will roll along a straight line and back without deviating from the line.*
5. *She will catch a large ball using both hands, 2 of 3 trials.*

Treatment Plan

CNS Preparation:
- *Initially keep room darkened, speak softly, gradually adding light as tolerated*
- *Slow rolling wrapped in blanket on trampoline*
- *Slow rocking on a title board (prone, supine or sidelying) or in a rocking chair*

Sensory Activities:
- *Apply lotion to body parts; wash face and arms with washcloth and warm water then dry with soft towel (these activities also relate to self-help skills)*
- *Make drawing with chalk on carpet, erase with both hands*

Gross Motor Activities:
• *Roll in carpeted barrel (to inhibit ATNR and total flexor patterns while facilitating body rotation); roll from one point to another*
• *Prone activities (begin with a wedge to support upper trunk); weight shift side to side while reaching for objects*
• *In sitting and/or kneeling, weight shift side to side with trunk rotation while moving game pieces or sorting objects.*

Fine Motor-Manipulative Activities:
• *Activities to achieve gross grasp/release using clay, Nerf balls*
• *Poke foam rubber chunks through small holes in coffee can cover; finger paint.*
• *Bat a suspended ball across mid-line from supine (watch for signs of over-arousal)*

Visual Skills:
• *Visual focus and tracking activities with flashlight on ceiling, on blackboard, etc.*

Behavior:
Keep non-essential environmental stimuli to a minimum; avoid topics which increase Cindy's excitatory level until her inhibitory mechanisms are in better balance; use verbal cues to keep on task and maintain attention.

Sample Report

Name: Dennis
Age: 7 years, 9 months
Test Date: September 10 and 16
Examiner: Eileen Richter, OTR

Pertinent Medical and Developmental History

Dennis was born two months premature, weighing 2 lbs, 8 ozs. He remained hospitalized for five months after birth. He has a history of ear and sinus infections, poor vision, and neglect by his biological mother who is intellectually handicapped. Dennis has been slow to reach developmental milestones and is receiving special education services.

Dennis' county social worker referred him for an occupational therapy evaluation to determine the need for intervention. He was seen for two one-hour evaluation sessions, one session taking place in his foster home. His foster mother expressed concern regarding his dislike of reading, printing, and coloring. She indicated interest in exercises or home activities which might benefit Dennis and requested recommendations which might be appropriately included in Dennis' Individual Education Program (IEP) goals/objectives.

Tests Administered

Sensorimotor Performance Analysis (SPA)

The SPA is a criterion-referenced assessment designed to evaluate the underlying sensorimotor components of a child's performance in several gross and fine motor tasks.

Miller Assessment for Preschoolers (MAP)

The MAP is a standardized instrument which, when used by an experienced therapist and augmented by supplemental clinical observations, evaluates the following developmental areas: neurological foundations; coordination; verbal, non-verbal, and complex tasks (the ability to use sensorimotor, verbal, and non-verbal skills to problem solve). Although the MAP standardization extends from 2.9 to 5.9 years, it is useful with older children who have severe developmental delays, providing a developmental overview and delineating patterns of strengths and weaknesses.

Observation

Includes additional observations made regarding behavior, quality of performance, responses to sensory input, and other subjective test items such as visual tracking, diadokokinesis, etc.

Behavior During Testing

Dennis is an engaging 7 year-old who can be outgoing at times yet reserved at other times. His best attending behavior was noted during table activities which were limited and structured, but his frustration tolerance was low at all times. He became distractible when faced with tasks which he perceived as difficult. During gross motor tasks, he had difficulty attending to the task and following direction. With support and encouragement, Dennis did attempt most of the test items presented.

Assessment Findings

I. *Sensory Development**

A. Awareness of Gravity and Motion: *The vestibular system gives basic necessary information for a stable, secure posture; large and fine motor skills; and eye control.*

Formal testing to determine the integrity of the vestibular system (Post-Rotary Nystagmus Test) was not administered. Functionally, Dennis seems to lack adequate vestibular processing to provide postural stability and security. His anti-gravity control is very poor, and balance reactions tend to be slow.

B. Awareness of Joint Position and Movement: *Contributes to stable posture and body scheme.*

Dennis demonstrates poor awareness and control of his own movements. He has difficulty grading his activity and movement as required in skilled motor tasks, relying therefore on total motor patterns and lots of movement. For example he is unable to maintain static postures for sitting or standing, instead using adjustment and extraneous motion to stay in one spot.

C. Awareness of Touch: *Gives basic information for body scheme, motor control and planning, and visual perception.*

Tactile items from the MAP indicate that Dennis is either not receiving adequate sensation from touch receptors or is not able to interpret the information properly. He was unable to identify objects through tactile exploration (stereognosis), particularly with his right hand. He also had some difficulty identifying which of his fingers had been touched when his vision was occluded. His foster mother reports that Dennis has a diminished response to pain.

D. Basic Visual Skills: *The first steps in visual perception of symbols.*

Dennis has significant visual problems which will make any visual-motor task difficult and laborious. Bilateral, occular coordination is jerky and dependent on head movement, particularly in his left visual field. His eyes have a tendency to wander. Although his right eye apparently has better acuity, he prefers to use his left eye from time to time.

E. Sensory Defensiveness or Dormancy: *Sometimes children may be overstimulated by or tend to seek more motion, touch, light, or visual input. Such responses interfere with sensory discrimination and attending behavior and can create avoidance behavior.*

Throughout testing, Dennis demonstrated discomfort with touch input from the examiner. He became more active and sometimes just dashed away. These are common responses indicative of tactile defensiveness. His behavior also indicates that he likes and needs lots of movement.

He was often better able to attend after short periods of rushing about the room.

II. *Motor Development*
(Posture and Movement)

Dennis has significant dysfunction in controlling basic postural movement patterns. As mentioned previously, he does not have normal control of flexion/extension patterns against gravity and therefore uses compensatory patterns. As a result, he has not developed head and trunk stability necessary as the foundation for skilled movement. Although he has rotational movement during rolling, he does not use rotation during upright, functional movement, and gross motor activity tends to lack smoothness, control, and gradation. In other words, he cannot grade his motor output to the requirements of the activity, i.e. he uses the same amount of effort and strength to pick up a hard, heavy object as to pick up a kitten.

Dennis has very poor cocontraction, using fixation for stability instead. This causes rigidity of posture, preventing the development of adequate balance responses and fluid, coordinated movement patterns. This can be seen carried over into fine motor tasks where shoulder elevation (fixation for stability) prevents fine controlled movements of the hands and fingers for such activities as drawing and cutting.

III. *Sensorimotor Development:*
The relationship of sensation to the body and its movements.

A. Bilateral Integration: *Awareness of each side of the body and its relationship to the other side as a basis for development of skilled hand coordination.*

Dennis has many problems which interfere with coordination of both sides of the body. He lacks reciprocal patterns between upper and lower extremities during crawling and other functional tasks. Rotation, which is a product of integration of the two sides of the body, is also deficient. He has difficulty coordinating his eyes for tracking and difficulty in using his hands efficiently on tasks which require both hands working together skillfully.

B. Motor Planning: *Thinking and planning unfamiliar movement patterns as opposed to automatic movements.*

Since he does not have the necessary sensorimotor development, Dennis has trouble in this area. He is unable to imitate simple postures or movement patterns, and he cannot quickly get a bead through a simple maze (MAP item) nor imitate simple tongue movements.

C. Visual Form and Space Perception: *Result of posture and eye control, perception of gravity, touch, and proprioception.*

Test scores on MAP items relating to visual perception indicate that Dennis has difficulty with figure-ground perception and puzzle completion as well as eye-hand coordination tasks.

IV. *Functional and Learning Activities: Result of Integration of Previous Sensory and Motor Abilities*

Considering Dennis' deficits in the basic foundational areas of sensorimotor development, it is not surprising that he dislikes printing or coloring. His sensory dysfunction contributes to distractibility; lack of trunk and postural stability makes fine motor tasks extremely difficult to achieve; and visual problems increase the difficulty of performing eye-hand coordination activities. (Most people do avoid tasks which put such demands on their limited abilities.) Dennis is also aware of and sensitive to failure.

Summary

Dennis exhibits signs of significant sensorimotor dysfunction and mild neurological abnormalities. These include mild choreoathetosis; associated reactions; poor coordination for slow motion and rapidly alternating movements (diadokokinesis); and oral dyspraxia (imitation of tongue movements). Sensory deficits include decreased tactile and pain awareness and discrimination; tactile defensiveness; inadequate gravity and proprioceptive responses; and poor visual perception. Motor dysfunction may be summarized as postural instability due to poor anti-gravity patterns and inadequate cocontraction which have led to abnormal compensatory fixation patterns; and incoordination resulting from sensory and neurological problems combined with the absence of normal stability.

Dennis has many strengths which can be emphasized in the educational process. With encouragement, he is willing to try and seems genuinely anxious to please. Test scores on the MAP show that his visual memory is good for simple sequencing and object memory as compared to children 5 years, 9 months. He also did fairly well with digit repetition which may be an indication that auditory memory is a strength.

Recommendations

Dennis could benefit from occupational therapy services designed to improve sensory processing and adaptive responses (motor output). Enclosed with this report is a *Treatment/Progress Profile*** which identifies appropriate objectives for treatment planning for Dennis. These objectives may also be used to develop an IEP to meet his needs in sensorimotor development and adaptive behavior.

Also enclosed are some simple activities which can be done at home to improve sensory responses and postural control. They should be done *in sequence* and repeated often. These activities can be a "family exercise program" with the family doing them together to make them more fun for Dennis. *These exercises are just a beginning and should be suppplimented with a regular therapy program to be effective.*

A number of group sensorimotor programs would be beneficial to Dennis (and perhaps other children in his class). One in particular requires a minimum of equipment and can be carried out by teachers in consultation with an occupational therapist. Should Dennis' teacher or therapist be interested, I would be happy to acquaint them with the program.

It has been a pleasure working with Dennis. If I can be of assistance in the future, don't hesitate to contact me.

Eileen W. Richter, MPH, OTR

---

*Description of assessment areas and terms were taken from the "St. Paul Schools Early Education Occupational Therapy Report" form developed by Mary Cowen, MS, OTR.
**Treatment/Progress Profile developed by Patricia Oetter, MA, OTR and Nancy Lawton-Shirley, OTR.

Sensorimotor Performance Analysis

Name _Dennis_
Birthdate _12/20/8C_
Date of Evaluation _9/10 ~ 16/87_

Age _7 yrs. 9 mos._
Evaluator _E. R._
Additional Information _____

Item A: Rolling

Won't lie down to roll _____ Will not roll _____

		Poor		Optimal
1.	Rolls both directions	1 lt___ rt___	3	(5)
2.	Motor planning	1 lt___ rt___	(3)	5
3.	Body righting	1 lt___ rt___	3	(5)
4.	Head righting a. prone b. supine c. lateral	1 (2) 1 (2) 1	3 (4) 3 5 (3)	5 5 5
5.	Asymmetrical tonic neck	(1) lt ✓ rt ✓	3	5
6.	Antigravity flexion	1 (2)	3	5
7.	Antigravity extension a. hips flexed b. knees flexed c. arms flexed	1 ___ ___ ___	3 (4)	5
8.	Becomes dizzy	1	3	(5)

Item B: Belly Crawling

Will not assume or maintain a prone position _____

Will not crawl fast _____

		Poor		Optimal
1.	Motor planning	1	(3)	5
2.	Hand position a. pulls with forearms not hands b. hands fisted c. fingertips only d. palms only e. uses whole hand to pull	1 ___ ___ ___ ___	3	(5) ✓
3.	Extremity lag	(1) lt ✓ rt ✓ UE LE	3	5
4.	Propulsion-feet & knees push	(1)	3	5
5.	Antigravity extension	(1)	3	5
6.	Prone head righting	1	(3)	5
7.	Upper trunk extension	(1)	3	5
8.	Lateral trunk movement	(1)	3	5
9.	Crawling pattern a. homolateral/ATNR b. homologous/STNR c. reciprocal	(1) ✓	3	5 ___ ___

Notes _Item C – Did not test._

Gets frustrated quickly

Item C: Bat the Ball from Hands and Knees

		Poor		Optimal
1.	Maintains 4-pt. position	1	3	5
2.	Eye tracking	1	3	5
3.	Visual avoiding reaction	1	3	5
4.	Crosses midline visually	1 lt___ rt___	3	5
5.	Crosses midline motorically	1 lt___ rt___	3	5
6.	Head righting	1	3	5
7.	Symmetrical tonic neck	1	3	5
8.	Hand position of support arm a. fisted b. fingertips only c. palms only d. whole hand flat	1 lt___ rt___ lt___ rt___ lt___ rt___ lt___ rt___	3	5
9.	Hand position of hitting arm a. fisted b. fingertips only c. palms only d. whole hand flat	1 lt___ rt___ lt___ rt___ lt___ rt___ lt___ rt___	3	5
10.	Maintains 3-pt. position	1 lt___ rt___	3	5
11.	Asymmetrical tonic neck	1 lt___ rt___	3	5
12.	Shoulder control	1 lt___ rt___	3	5
13.	Eye hand coordination	1 lt___ rt___	3	5

Item D: Kneeling Balance

Will not assume kneeling position _____

		Poor		Optimal
1.	Assumes kneeling	1	(3)	5
2.	Maintains kneeling position	1	(3)	5
3.	Hip stability	1	(2)	3 5
4.	Tolerates movement	1	3	(5)
5.	Lateral head righting	1	(3)	5
6.	Trunk righting	1	(3)	5
7.	Extremity righting a. upper extremities b. lower extremities	1 lt___ rt___ lt___ rt___	(3)	5
8.	Protective extension	1 lt___ rt___	3 (4)	5
9.	Body rotation	1	3 (4)	5
10.	Antigravity extension	1	(3)	5
11.	Antigravity flexion	1	(3)	5
12.	Symmetrical tonic neck	1 (2)	3	5
13.	Asymmetrical tonic neck	1 lt___ rt___	3 (4)	5

Item E: Pellets in Bottle

	Poor		Optimal
1. Trunk stability	1 (2) 3		5
2. Trunk posture	1 (3)		5
3. Head position	1	3	(5)
a. mid-position	lt___ rt___		
b. flexed	1	3	(5)
c. extended	1	3	(5)
4. Uses unilateral reach	1	3	(5)
5. Grasp adequate for age	(1)	3	5
a. palmer grasp			
b. superior palmer grasp	___		
c. lateral pinch	___		
d. inferior pincer grasp	___		
e. radial digital grasp	✓		
f. forefinger pinch			
6. Mouths or bangs bottle	1	3	(5)
7. Avoiding reactions	1	3	(5)
8. Puts pellets in bottle	1	3	(5)
9. Picks pellets up in sequence	1	3	(5)
10. Changes hand at mid-line	1	(3)	5
11. Preferred hand _____	1	(3)	5
12. Dumps pellets out	1	3	(5)
13. Tremor	1	3	(5)
14. Associated reactions	1	3 (4)	5

Item F: Pencil and Paper Task

	Poor		Optimal
1. Trunk stability	1	(3)	5
2. Trunk posture	1	(3)	5
3. Head position	1	3	(5)
a. mid-position	lt___ rt___		
b. flexed	1	3	(5)
c. extended	1	3	(5)
4. Differentiates ends of pencil	1	3	(5)
5. Positions paper to body center	1	3	(5)
	lt___ rt___		
6. Stabilizes paper with one hand	1	3	(5)
7. Pencil position	(1)	3	5
a. gross grasp (fist)			
b. lateral pinch	✓		
c. radial-digital pinch	___		
d. avoids placing fingertips on pencil	___		
e. thumb/forefinger opposition, pencil resting on 2nd finger			
8. Forearm position	1	(3)	5
9. Grip strength	1	3 (4)	5
hypotonic			
hypertonic	✓		
10. Drawing pressure	1	(3)	5
excessively heavy	✓		
excessively light			
11. Preferred hand (lt___ rt___)			
a. switches during testing	1	3	(5)
b. draws across body mid-line	1	3	(5)
	lt___ rt___		
12. Imitates strokes	1	3	(5)
a. vertical			
b. circular	✓		
c. scribbles	✓		
d. bangs/mouths pencil	___		
13. Copies			
a. circle	1	3	(5)
b. cross	1	3	(5)
14. Upper extremity movement	1	(3)	5
a. primarily shoulder			
b. elbow/forearm	✓		
c. wrist/finger	✓		
15. Associated movements	1 (2)	3	5
16. Tremor	1	3	(5)

Item G: Scissor Task

	Poor		Optimal
1. Trunk stability	1 (2)	3	5
2. Trunk posture	1 (2)	3	5
3. Head position	(1)	3	5
a. mid-position	lt ✓ rt___		
b. flexed	1	(3)	5
c. extended	1	3	(5)
4. Shoulder position	(1)	3	5
5. Forearm holding paper	(1)	3	5
a. pronated	✓		
b. supinated			
6. Hand grip holding paper	1	(3)	5
a. hypotonic	✓		
b. hypertonic	___		
7. Forearm cutting paper	1	3	(5)
a. pronated	___		
b. supinated			
8. Wrist position during cutting	(1)	3	5
a. flexion	✓		
b. extension	___		
c. ulnar deviation	___		
9. Hand cutting paper	1	(3)	5
a. lateral pinch	✓		
b. forefinger pinch	___		
c. thumb/hand opposition			___
10. Unused fingers-cutting hand	1 (2)	3	5
11. Visual orienting	1	3	(5)
12. Cut is continuous/smooth	(1)	3	5
13. Straight line is accurate	1 (2)	3	5
14. Curved line is accurate	1 (2)	3	5
15. Preferred hand	1	(3)	5
lt ✓ rt___			
16. Tremor	1	3	(5)
17. Associated reactions	(1)	3	5

Reflex Activity Assessment

	REFLEX OR RESPONSE	Poor-Optimal		
Spinal	TACTILE DEFENSIVENESS	P	F	A
BRAIN STEM	ASYMMETRICAL TONIC NECK-RIGHT	P	F	A
	AYMMETRICAL TONIC NECK-LEFT	P	F	A
	SYMMETRICAL TONIC NECK	P	F	A
	ANTIGRAVITY FLEXION	P	F	A
	ANTIGRAVITY EXTENSION	P	F	A
	ASSOCIATED REACTIONS	P	F	A
MID BRAIN	NECK RIGHTING	P	F	A
	BODY RIGHTING	A	F	P
	HEAD RIGHTING-PRONE	A	F	P
	HEAD RIGHTING-SUPINE	A	F	P
AUTO-MATIC	STARTLE	P	F	A
	LANDAU	P	F	A
	PROTECTIVE EXTENSION	A	F	P

	EQUILIBRIUM REACTIONS	RT.	LT.
COR-TICAL	PRONE HEAD RTG.	A F P	A F P
	SUPINE TRUNK RTG.	A F P	A F P
	SITTING PROTECTIVE EXT.	A F P	A F P
	KNEELING EXTREMITIES	A F P	A F P

Notes *Not tested for Reflex Activity.*

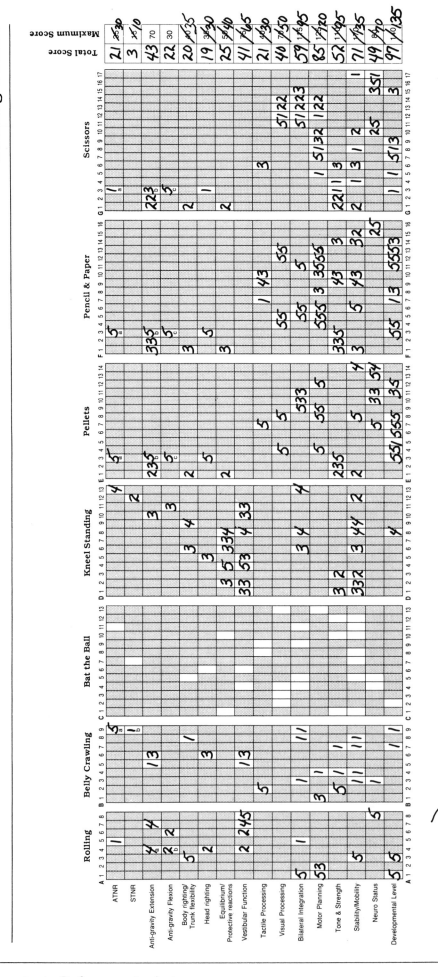

Name Dennis   Age 7¾

Evaluator E. Richter   Case Manager

Date 9-87

Appendices

Ayres, A. J. (1964). Tactile functions: Their relation to hyperactive behavior. *American Journal of Occupational Therapy, 18,* 6-11.

Ayres, A. J. (1972). *Sensory integration and learning disorders.* Los Angeles: Western Psychological Services, Inc.

Ayres, A. J. (1974). *The development of sensory integrative theory and practice: A collection of the works of A. Jean Ayres.* Dubuque, IA: Kendall/Hunt. (Factor analytic studies 1965-1974 are in this collection.)

Ayres, A. J. (1985). *Developmental dypraxia and adult onset dyspraxia.* Torrance, CA: Sensory Integration International.

Bishop, B. (1974). Vibratory stimulation: Part I. Neurophysiology of motor responses evoked by vibratory stimulation. *Physical Therapy, 54,* 1273-1282.

Bishop, B. (1975a). Vibratory stimulation: Part II. Vibratory stimulation as an evaluation tool. *Physical Therapy, 55,* 28-34.

Bishop, B. (1975b). Vibratory stimulation: Part III. Possible applications of vibration in treatment of motor dysfunctions. *Physical Therapy, 55,* 139-143.

Bobath, K. (1985). *Abnormal postural reflex activity caused by brain lesions* (3rd ed.). Rockville, MD: Aspen Publications.

Bosma, J. F. (1967). *Symposium on oral sensation and perception.* Springfield, IL: Charles C. Thomas.

Bundy, A. C., & Fisher, A. G. (1981). The relationship of prone extension to other vestibular functions. *American Journal of Occupational Therapy, 35,* 782-787.

Cermak, S., Coster, W., & Drake C. (1980). Representational and nonrepresentational gestures in boys with learning disabilities. *American Journal of Occupational Therapy, 34,* 19-26.

Cermak, S., Quintero, E. J., & Cohen, P. M. (1980). Developmental age trends in crossing the body midline in normal children. *American Journal of Occupational Therapy, 34,* 313-319.

Clark, D. (1985). The vestibular system: an overview of structure and function. *Physical & Occupational Therapy in Pedicatrics, 5* (2/3), 5-32.

Clark, F. (1983). Research on the neuropathophysiology of autism and its implications for occupational therapy. *Occupational Therapy Journal of Research, 3,* 3-22.

Conrad, K. E., Cermak, S. A., & Drake, C. (1983). Differentiation of praxis among children. *American Journal of Occupational Therapy, 37,* 466-473.

Degangi, G. A. (1982). Relationship of vestibular responses and developmental functions in high risk infants. *Physical & Occupational Therapy in Pediatrics, 2*(2/3), 35-49.

Eccles, J. C. (1966). The understanding of the brain. New York: McGraw-Hill.

Eviatar, L. (1974). The maturation of neurovestibular responses in infants. *Developmental Medicine and Child Neurology, 16,* 435-446.

Fisher, A. G., Mixon, J., & Herman, R. (1986). Validity of the clinical diagnosis of vestibular dysfunction. *Occupational Therapy Journal of Research, 6,* 3-20.

Goodgold-Edwards, S. A. (1984). Motor learning as it relates to the development of skilled motor behavior: A review of the literature, *Physical & Occupational Therapy in Pediatrics, 4*(4), 5-18.

Harlow, H. F., & Harlow, M. K. (1962). Social deprivation in monkeys. *Scientific American, 207,* 136-146.

Harris, S. R. (1981). Neuropathology in cerebral palsy. *Physical & Occupational Therapy in Pediatrics, 1* (4), 45-52.

Harris, N. (1981). Duration and quality of the prone extension position in four-, six-, and eight-year-old normal children. *American Journal of Occupational Therapy, 35,* 26-30.

Holt, K. (Ed.). (1975). *Movement and child development. Clinics in developmental medicine, No. 55.* Philadelphia: J. B.

Lippincott Co.

Magoun, H. W. (1981). *The waking brain.* Springfield, IL: Charles C. Thomas.

Mason, W. A., & Berkson, G. (1975). Effects of maternal mobility on the development of rocking and other behaviors in rhesus monkeys: A study with artificial mothers. *Developmental Psychobiology, 8,* 197-211.

Mayberry, W. (1985). Ocular pursuit in mentally retarded, cerebral palsied and learning disabled children, *American Journal of Occupational Therapy, 39,* 589-95.

Montgomery, P. C. (1985). Assessment of vestibular function in children, *Physical & Occupational Therapy in Pediatrics.* 5(2/3), 33-55.

Moore, J. C. (1973). *Concepts from the Neurobehavioral Sciences.* Dubuque, IA: Kendall/Hunt.

Moore, J. C. (1984). The golgi tendon organ: A review and update. *American Journal of Occupational Therapy, 38,* 227-236,

Montague, A. (1971). *Touching: The human significance of the skin.* New York: Columbia University press.

Noback, C. R., & Demarest, R. I (1975). *The human nervous system.* New York: McGraw-Hill Book Co.

Northwestern University Special Therapeutic Exercise Project. (1967). Proceedings: An exploratory and analytical survey of therapeutic exercise. Northwestern University special therapeutic exercise project. *American Journal of Physical Medicine, 46*(1).

Ottenbacher, K. J. (1982). Vestibular processing dysfunction in children with emotional and behavioral disorders: A review. *Physical & Occupational Therapy in Pediatrics, 2*(1), 3-12.

Ottenbacher, K. J. (1980). Excessive postrotary nystagmus duration in learning disabled children. *American Journal of Occupational Therapy, 34,* 40-44.

Ottenbacher, K. J., & Short, M. A. (1979). Association between nystagmus hypo responsivity and behavioral problems in learning-disabled children. *American Journal of Occupational Therapy, 33,* 317-322.

Ottenbacher, K. J., Watson, P. J., Short, M. A., & Biderman, M. D. (1979). Nystagmus and ocular fixation difficulties in learning-disabled children. *American Journal of Occupational Therapy, 33,* 317-322.

deQuiros, J., & Schrager, O. L. (1977). *Neuropsychological fundamentals in learning disabilities.* San Rafael, CA: Academic Therapy.

Petri, J. L., & Anderson, M. E. (1980). Eye and head movements in reading-disabled and normal children. *American Journal of Occupational Therapy, 34,* 801-808.

Purpura, D. P. (1974). Dendritic spine dysgenesis and mental retardation. *Science, 186,* 1126-1128.

Saint-Anne Dargassies, S. (1977). *Neurological development in the full term and premature infant.* New York: Excerpta Medica.

Shuer, J., Clark, F., & Azen, S. P. (1980). Vestibular functions in mildly mentally retarded adults. *American Journal of Occupational Therapy, 34,* 664-670.

Steinbeck, T. M. (1986). Purposeful activity and performance. *American Journal of Occupational Therapy, 40,* 529-534.

Stilwell, J. M., Crowe, T. L., & McCallum, L. W. (1978). Postrotary nystagmus duration as a function of communication disorders. *American Journal of Occupational Therapy, 32,* 222-228.

Umphred, D. A. (1985). *Neurological rehabilitation.* St. Louis, MO: C. V. Mosby Co.

Van Sant, A. F. (1987). Concepts of neural organization and movement. In B. H. Connolly & P. C. Montgomery (Eds.), *Therapeutic exercise in developmental disabilities.* Chattanooga, TN: Chattanooga Publishing.

Developmental Milestones And Their Significance

The Fetus
(12 Weeks Gestation - Term)

Significant Achievements
- Develops every human movement pattern by 20 weeks gestation.
- Demonstrates sensory functions by responding to touch (7 weeks gestation); gravity (especially for birth presentation); orienting to sounds (27 weeks); and light (29 weeks).

Typical Sensorimotor Behaviors
- *Extremely active!* Progresses rapidly from disorganized flexor-extensor jerks (10 weeks)to extension with scissoring to thrusting patterns.
- Sucking and swallowing by 15 weeks.
- Head rotation by 15 weeks.
- Reciprocal and symmetrical limb movements by 17 weeks.

Relevance for Future Development
- The fetus is preparing to participate as a partner in the birthing process: getting into position, "springing off," etc.
- Has well-established suck/swallow for feeding at birth.
- Has begun to develop attention and habituation skills for learning.
- Has established crawling patterns and automatic walking, evident at birth.

The Newborn
(0 - 1 Week)

Typical Sensorimotor Behaviors
- *Gross Motor:* Nonreflexive activity is gross and random. Flexor tone (physiological flexion) predominates. Reacts to sudden changes with total body.
- *Prone:* Turns head side to side; body floppy and frog-like; hips and knees flexed; buttocks up.
- *Sitting:* Head falls forward and back; head lags when pulled to sit
- *Fine Motor:* Hands fisted.

- *Reflexes* (Primary Motor Patterns): Grasp (plantar and palmar) Moro, startle, automatic stepping, flexor withdrawal, traction response, ATNR, STNR, crossed extension, placing reaction, neck righting, extensor thrust, rooting, sucking, etc.
- *Perceptual*: Sees patterns, light and dark, focuses 8 inches, can locate and discriminate sounds, discriminates tastes.
- *Speech*: Smiles spontaneously, cries, animal-like vocalizations.

Relevance for Future Development
- Protection: Most of the neonate's motor behavior is in the nature of withdrawal responses designated to protect the organism from harmful stimuli.
- Survival: Rooting and sucking provide the necessary behavior for nourishment; establishes a bond with caretaker.

One-Two Months
(4 -10 Weeks)

Significant Achievements
- Stabilization of bodily functions.
- Increasing control of head in all positions.
- Coordination of eye movement.
- Hands start to open.

Typical Sensorimotor Behaviors
- *Supine*: Head and extremity posture predominantly asymmetrical (ATNR).
- *Prone*: Head in mid-position, can hold at 45 degree angle for a short time.
- *Sitting*: With support, head can be held erect though it bobs.
- *Fine Motor:* Desire to grasp is shown by excitement and generalized body movement; incidental touching leads to fisted swiping; may begin to contemplate hand.
- *Perceptual:* Coordinates eye movements and tracks objects past mid-line; clearly discriminates among voices, people, tastes, proximity, and object size.
- *Speech:* Coos.

Relevance for Future Development

- The ATNR provides the opportunity for the infant to spend much time focusing on his hands, which is the beginning of eye-hand coordination (and coordination of eye movement).
- Decreasing grasp reflex and open hand pave the way for voluntary grasp.
- Upper trunk and head stability are increasing (through weight shift and development of extensor muscles) in readiness for sitting.

Three-Four Months
(16 Weeks)

Significant Achievements

- Overcoming gravity in the head region in prone position. Mechanisms acting to bring about this stage:
    1. Labyrinthine righting reactions and "swimming movements" in prone.
    2. Disappearance of the ATNR and beginning of the Landau.
    3. Weight shift down spinal column toward abdomen.

Typical Sensorimotor Behaviors

- *Prone:* Supports on forearms, head/chest up, face vertical. Kicks reflexively, alternating and sometimes together. One arm is often more flexed than the other, which makes equilibrium unstable, exercises extensor muscles, and causes diagonal weight shift.
- *Supine:* Head usually in the mid-line, limbs symmetrical. Cannot yet lift head from supine; better control of anti-gravity flexion.
- *Sitting:* When pulled to sitting, the head lags only slightly. Held sitting, the head is erect and steady but is set forward. Back rounded only in lumbar region.
- *Standing:* Held standing, briefly sustains fraction of weight; legs extending intermittently and rising on toes. May lift one foot, and toes tend to flex (grasp).
- *Hand use* and eye-*hand behavior:*
    1. Beginnings of voluntary grasp (as opposed to reflex grasp).
    2. Supine: Hands engage near mouth or chest and are more open, with fingers only slightly flexed. May clutch at clothing or blanket and pull up over face. Arms are activated when an object is suspended above: Reaches toward the object with both arms in unison, but contact is accidental. When a rattle or ring is placed in his hand, he will retain and regard it and bring it to his mouth. Eyes will follow an object through an arc of 180 degrees.
    3. Prone: "Puppy position," receives tactile and pressure stimuli on the heel of his hand, which helps him to open hands and begin exploration with fingers, scratches the surface.
    4. Held in sitting: Looks at objects and arms activate. Child will look at object, at his hand, and then back at object as though "measuring the distance." Hands may not yet obey eyes for reach and grasp although he may touch the object.
- *Speech:* Coos, makes some vowel sounds, is aware of and interested in own voice. Spontaneous social smile and more differentiation of facial expression. Shows interest by overall pattern of straining whole body forward with associated rapid, heavy breathing.

Relevance for Future Development:
Prone "puppy position":
1. Strengthens spinal extensors (in preparation for sitting).
2. Weight-bearing on arms strengthens fixators for future reaching and lifting movements and gives the postural basis for developing hand use.
3. Shifting weight to one arm increases support tone in that arm (in preparation for freeing other arm to reach and grasp). Also marks beginning of equilibrium responses in head and upper trunk in prone.
4. Face vertical with a widened horizon (beginning of spatial orientation).
5. Legs more extended: Prepares for Landau response.
6. Development of beginning equilibrium in prone and disappearance of ATNR in supine affords control between these two positions — sidelying emerging (in preparation for control of rolling).

- *Supine:* Disappearance of the ATNR in supine affords control of rolling (in preparation for transfer and bimanual activities).

Six-Seven Months
(30 Weeks)

Significant Achievements
- Ability to sit when placed or propped. Begins to free arms for use of both hands together; develops rolling. Mechanisms acting to bring about this stage.
  1. Inhibition of Moro (although this reflex had almost disappeared in the "puppy" stage, it reappeared briefly when mother began placing infant in sitting position).
  2. Labyrinthine righting reaction in prone progressing caudal-ward: The Landau reinforced by optical righting.
  3. Modification of neck righting reaction. Beginning rotation between thorax and pelvis (beginning of body righting reactions).
  4. Equilibrium control in prone.
  5. Protective extension of arms forward ("forward parachute").
  6. Legs undergoing inhibitory phase: Less reflex kicking.

Typical Sensorimotor Behaviors
- *Prone:* Head well-lifted and can lift legs high in extension. Legs are quieter and "amphibian reaction" can be elicited. Tries to pivot on abdomen. Can reach with one arm. May lift onto hands and knees (using STNR), but cannot yet rock or creep.
- *Supine:* Lifts head (wants to sit up). Labyrin-thine righting. Pulls extended legs up high; brings feet to mouth. May not like supine and will roll immediately to prone.
- *Sitting:* Cannot yet assume sitting position independently, but must be placed in or pulled to sitting. Balances briefly then props forward on hands. Rocks back and forth (as if searching for center of gravity).
- *Standing:* Held standing, sustains most of weight and bounces actively. May rock pelvis as if trying to step, but reflex stepping has disappeared and volitional stepping has not yet emerged.
- *Hand Use and Eye-Hand Behavior:*
  1. Has mastered grasp; grasps compulsively and brings objects to mouth.
  2. Former bilateral approach to objects is becoming unilateral; when sitting supported, reaches and grasps object with one hand then transfers it. Grasp has changed from ulnar-palmar to radial-palmar.
  3. Presented a pellet, cannot secure it with hand, but "rakes" at it with fingers.
  4. Constantly inspects objects with eyes, hands, and mouth. He feels, rotates, mouths, transfers, inspects, bangs, and drops, then resecures object to begin the process again.
- *Speech:* Beginning labial (lip) sounds, "m-m-m," "pa-pa," "ba-ba." Begins to combine vowel sounds (diphthongs). Chewing begins (as opposed to biting) which involves slight rotary motion of mandible and shifting of food from side to side with the tongue.

Relevance for Future Development
- Developing control between prone and supine in rolling is in preparation for:
  1. Pushing to sitting ("ventral push").
  2. Rotation necessary for equilibrium responses in sitting.
- Labyrinthine righting in supine strengthens abdominals for control in sitting.
- Pulling feet to mouth strengthens abdominals, prepares for independent sitting.
- Landau: Further strengthening of extensors (in preparation for completely erect sitting and for standing).
- Bouncing and bearing weight on feet and diminishing reflex activity of legs (in preparation for control in standing).
- Behavior with objects affords visual, tactual, auditory, and gustatory stimulation necessary for perceptual growth.
- Lip closure achieved in forming labial sounds marks the beginning of drooling control.

Eight-Ten Months
(42 Weeks)

Significant Achievements
• Mastery of sitting which "emancipates" the hands. Can creep and pull to standing. Mechanisms acting to bring about this stage:
  1. Complete inhibition of reflex activity in the legs.
  2. Labyrinthine and body righting reactions which allow child to assume sitting and return to prone.
  3. Protective extension to front (5-6 months), side (6-8 months), and back (8-10 months) which allows baby complete freedom in sitting.
  4. Strong Landau.

Typical Sensorimotor Behaviors
• *Prone:* Spent last two months getting to all fours and finding center of gravity by rocking. May also rock on hands and feet ("bear-walking" or "Plantigrade position") and sometimes a combination, i.e. one foot, one knee. Can pivot on abdomen, pull forward with arms, and creep. (Note: A small percentage of infants do not creep or bear-walk, but "hitch in sitting.")
• *Sits* alone indefinitely and completely erect. Can twist and turn, bend over, and regain sitting. Goes easily from sitting to prone (all fours) and back by "vaulting" over one leg. No longer must overbalance forward as child has upper extremity propping to the sides and back.
• *Standing:* Pulls to standing usually through half-kneeling. At first, may not lower himself with control, but may fall backward to sit or may stand and cry for help. Learns to get down, often by letting go with one hand and turning sideways to reach floor with free hand.
• *Hand Use and Eye-Hand Behavior:* Characterized by poking and exploring third dimension with index finger "forefinger to fore."
  1. Grasp: Radial-digital (as opposed to palmar). Thumb has become actively involved (pincer grasp). Interest directed to small objects. Can pick up pellet, but cannot yet insert into bottle.
  2. Relates two cubes; holds, mouths ball, but release is not perfected.
  3. Holds own bottle, finger feeds, plays pat-a-cake, waves "bye bye."
• *Speech:* One or two simple words with double syllables ("mama"); understands "no"; and likes to make funny noises such as coughing, clicking tongue, vibrating lips. Begins imitating sounds and copying gestures. Stress (8-10 months) of learning to stand and teething may increase drooling.

Relevance for Future Development
• Strength of Landau encourages full weight-bearing with heels down.
• Beginning standing indicates equilibrium in sitting and all fours is almost perfected which allows exploration with body and hands (begins to learn how his body moves in space).
• Creeping or bear-walking prepares for reciprocation in walking.
• Relating of two cubes prepares for ability to build a tower (once release becomes perfected).

Ten-Twelve Months
(52 Weeks)

Significant Achievements
• Cruising: Formative period for abilities which will not be complete in organization until 15-18 months. The mechanisms acting to bring about this stage and subsequent stages are increasingly mature equilibrium reactions.

Typical Sensorimotor Behaviors
• *Locomotion:*
  1. Uses both quadruped/biped methods; prefers perfected quadruped for "important projects and exploration" as it is faster and more secure.
  2. Begins independent walking between 12-15 months, first laterally. Toddler gait is wide-based and characterized by picking leg up high in flexion-external rotation, thrusting it out and down. Arms are outstretched or in "high-guard" position.

- *Prehension:* Combination of mature/immature skills with increased precision in grasp, but precision in release continues to be difficult.
    1. Can release cube into cup, but cannot build tower of two cubes.
    2. Cannot insert a pellet in a bottle.
    3. Offers ball on request, but does not release it.
- *Speech:* Understanding of language increases, but expansion of vocabulary slows down when he learns to walk. Responds to music and rhythm. Begins to develop perception of geometric form, number, and spatial relationships.

Relevance for Future Development
- Cruising: Strengthens hip abductors and rotator cuff (in preparation for walking with one hand held).
- Coordinated, quick, reciprocal creeping prepares for reciprocal arm-swing in erect locomotion.
- Perceptual skills are practised. Begins to scribble. At 15 months, will attempt to turn doorknobs.

Eighteen Months
(74 Weeks)

Typical Sensorimotor Behaviors
- *Walks* well, seldom falls. Creeping has been discarded. Can use hands while walking (age of the pull toy). Runs stiffly. Squats during play.
- *Equilibrium* in walking is developing and will continue to develop for another 18 months. At three years, child will stand on one foot and alternate feet on stairs.
- *Release* becomes more precise:
    1. Can build tower of 3-4 cubes.
    2. Inserts pellet in bottle and dumps it out.
- *Vocabulary* of about ten words. Understands pictures and symbols. Likes picture books and points to pictures. Turns two to three pages of book at a time. Scribbles and imitates a stroke.

Relevance for Future Development
- Righting reactions dominate child's movement. Rolls over, climbs to feet and onto furniture compulsively. He is "motor driven," practising (endlessly) skills, especially rotary components (which prepare him for mature equilibrium in all planes).

——————— *References* ———————

Blankenstein, M., Dehaas, J., & Welberger, U. (1975). *The Development of the infant: The first year of life in photographs.* London: Heinemann Medical Books, Ltd.

Bly, L. (1983). *Components of normal movement during the first year of life and abnormal motor development.* Chicago: NDT Association.

Bobath, B., & Bobath. K. (1975). *Motor development in the different types of cerebral palsy.* London: Heinemann Medical Books, Ltd.

Brazelton, T. B. (1984). (2nd ed.). *Neonatal Behavioral Assessment Scale. Clinics in Developmental Medicine, No. 50.* Philadelphia: J. B. Lippincott.

Gilfoyle, E., Grady, A., & Moore, J. C. (1981). *Children adapt.* Thorofare, N. J.: Charles J. Slack.

Gesell, A., & Armatruda, C. S. (1974). *Developmental diagnosis.* New York: Paul B. Hoeber.

Lohrey, B. (1972, January-March). *Pediatric Care Course.* Adaptation of material presented at Pediatric Care Course. San Francisco, CA.

McGraw, M. (1966). *The neuromuscular maturation of the human infant.* New York: Hafner Publishing Co.

Milani-Comparetti, A., & Gidoni, E. A. (1967). Pattern analysis of motor development and its disorders. *Developmental Medicine & Child Neurology, 9,* 625-630.

Milani-Comparetti, A. (1981). The neurophysiological and clinical implications of studies on fetal motor behavior. *Seminars in Perinatology, 5,* 183-189.

Pieper, A. (1963) *Cerebral function in infancy and childhood.* New York: Consultants Bureau.

Developmental Issues

Andre-Thomas, Chesni, Y., & Saint-Anne Dargassies S. (1960). *Neurological examination of the infant. Clinics in developmental medicine, No. 1*. Philadelphia: J. B. Lippincott Co.

Ayres, A. J. (1979). Sens*ory integration and the child*. Los Angeles: Western Psychological Services.

Blankenstein, M., Welberger,U., & Dehaas, J. (1975). *The development of the infant: The first year of life in photographs*. London: William Heinemann Medical Books, Ltd.

Bly, L. (1983). *Components of normal movement during the first year of life and abnormal motor development*. Chicago: NDT Association.

Bobath, B., & Bobath, K. (1966). *Motor development in the different types of cerebral palsy*. New York: William Heinemann Medical Books, Ltd.

Bobath, K., & Bobath B. (1962). An analysis of the development of standing and walking patterns in patients with cerebral palsy. *Physiotherapy, 48*, 144-148.

Bradley, R. H. & Caldwell, B. M. (1979). Home environment and cognitive development in the first two years. *Developmental Psychology, 15*(3) 246-250.

Brazelton, T. (1969). *Infants and mothers*. New York: Delta Publishing Co., Inc.

Brazelton, T. (1974). *Toddlers and parents*. New York: Delacorte Press/Seymour Lawrence.

Brazelton, T. (1984). *Neonatal behavioral assessment scale. Clinics in developmental medicine, No. 88* (2nd ed). Philadelphia: J. B. Lippincott Co.

Caplan, F. (1971). *The first twelve months of life*. New York: Grosset & Dunlap.

Caplan, F. (1974). *The second twelve months of life*. New York: Grosset & Dunlap.

Chase, R. A., & Rubin, R. R. (1979). *The first wondrous year*. New York: Collier Books.

Cohen, S. E., & Beckwith, L. (1976). Maternal language in infancy. *Developmental Psychology, 12*(4), 371-372.

Drillien, C. M. (1964). *The growth and development of the prematurely born infant*. Baltimore: Williams & Wilkins.

Drillien, C. M., & Drummond, M. B. (1977). *Neurodevelopmental problems in early childhood: Assessment and management*. Philadelphia: J. B. Lippincott.

Dubowitz, L. & Dubowitz, V., & Goldberg, C. (1970). Clinical assessment of gestational age in the newborn infant. *Journal of Pediatrics, 77*(1), 1-10.

Easton, T. A. (1972). On the normal use of reflexes. *American Scientist, 60*, 591-593.

Elliott, J. M., & Connolly K. J. (1984). A classification of manipulative hand movements. *Developmental Medicine and Child Neurology, 5*, 283-296.

Erhardt, R. (1974). Sequential levels in development of prehension. *American Journal of Occupational Therapy, 28*, 592-596.

Erickson, M. (1976). *Assessment and management of developmental changes in children*. St. Louis, MO: C. V. Mosby Company.

Gesell, A., & Armatruda, C. S. (1974). *Developmental diagnosis* (3rd ed.). New York: Paul B. Hoeber.

Gilfoyle, E., Grady, A., & Moore, J. C. (1981). *Children Adapt*. Thorofare, NJ.: Charles B. Slack.

Halvorson, H. M. (1931). Study of prehension in infants. *Genetic Psychological Monographs, 10*, 107-285.

Hoskins, T. S., & Squires, J. E. (1973). Developmental assessment: A test for gross motor and reflex development. *Physical Therapy, 53*, 117-126.

Humphrey, T. (1969). Postnatal repetition of human prenatal activity sequences with some suggestion of their neuroanatomical basis. In R. S. Robinson (Ed.), *Brain & early behavior: Development in the fetus and infant*. New York: Academic Press.

Ianniruberto, A. & Tajani, E. (1981). Ultrasonographic study of fetal movements. *Seminars in Perinatology, 5*, 175-181.

Illingworth, R. S. (1971). *The development of the infant and young child, normal and abnormal* (4th ed.). Baltimore: Williams & Wilkins Co.

Klat (1967a). Pattern analysis of motor development and its disorders. *Developmental Medicine and Child Neurology, 9,* 625-630.

Milani-Comparetti, A., & Gidoni, E. A. (1967b). Routine developmental examination in normal and retarded children. *Developmental Medicine and Child Neurology, 9,* 631-638.

Nilsson, L. (1965). *A child is born: The drama of life before birth.* New York: Del Publishing Company, Inc.

Prechtl, H. (Ed.). (1984). *Continuity of neural functions from prenatal to postnatal life. Clinics in developmental medicine, No. 94,* Philadelphia: J. B. Lippincott, 1984.

Robert, D. (1983). Effect of gestational age on neuromotor development of pre-term infants, *Physical & Occupational Therapy in Pediatrics, 3*(2), 23-42.

Sostek, A. M. (1978). Infant scales in the pediatric setting: The Brazelton neonatal assessment scale and the Carey infant temperament questionaire. *Journal of Pediatric Psychology, 3,* 113-121.

Stone, J., Smith, H., & Murphy (Eds.). (1973). *The competent infant.* New York: Basic Books.

Twitchell, T. E. (1965). Normal motor development. *Physical Therapy, 45,* 419-423.

Uzgiris U., & Hunt, J. (1975). *Assessment in infancy.* Chicago: University of Illinois Press.

Wachs, T., & DeRemer, P. (1978). Adaptive behavior and Uzgiris-Hunt scale performance in young children, developmentally disabled children. *American Journal of Mental Deficiency, 83,* 171-176.

Reflexes/Postural Responses

Ayres, A. J. (1972). *Sensory integration and learning disabilities*, Los Angeles: Western Psychological Services.

Bigsby, R. (1983). Reaching and ATNR in pre-term and full-term infants. *Physical & Occupational Therapy in Pediatrics*, 3(4), 25-42.

Bobath, K. (1985). *Abnormal postural reflex activity caused by brain lesions* (3rd Ed.). Rockville, MD: Aspen Publishers.

Coryell, J., Henderson, A., & Liederman, J. (1982). Factors influencing the asymmetrical tonic neck reflex in normal infants. *Physical & Occupational Therapy in Pediatrics*, 2(2/3), 51-65.

Easton, T. A. (1972). On the normal use of reflexes. *American Scientist*, 60, 591-593.

Fiorenino, M. R. (1981). *A basis for sensorimotor development - normal and abnormal*. Springfield, IL: Charles C. Thomas.

Fiorentino, M. R. (1976). *Reflex testing methods for evaluating CNS development*. Springfield, IL: Charles C. Thomas.

Fisher, A., & Bundy, A. (1982). Equilibrium reactions in normal children and in boys with sensory integrative dysfunction. *Occupational Therapy Journal of Research*, 2, 171-183.

Haley, S. M. (1986). Postural reactions in infants with Down Syndrome: Relationship to motor milestones, development, and age. *Physical Therapy*, 66, 17-22.

Haley, S. M. (1986). Sequential analyses of postural reactions in nonhandicapped infants. *Physical Therapy*, 66, 531-536.

Halverson, H. M. (1936). Complications of the early grasping reaction. *Psychological Monographs*, 47, 47-63.

Halverson, H. M. (1937). Studies of the grasp response in early infancy. *Journal of Genetic Psychology*, 51, 371-449.

Izraelevitz, T. A., Fisher, A., & Bundy, M. S. (1985). Equilibrium reactions in preschoolers, *Occupational Therapy Journal of Research*, 5, 154-169.

Ingram, T. (1962). Clinical significance of the infantile feeding reflexes, *Developmental Medicine and Child Neurology*, 4, 159-169.

Paine, R. S. (1964). Evolution of postural reflexes in normal infants and in the presence of chronic brain syndromes. *Neurology*, 4, 1036-1048.

Paine, R. S. (1964). The evaluation of infantile postural reflexes in the presence of chronic brain syndromes. *Developmental Medicine and Child Neurology*, 6, 345-361.

Parmenter, C. L. (1975). The asymmetrical tonic neck reflex in normal first and third grade children. *American Journal of Occupational Therapy*, 29, 463-468.

Parmenter, C. L. (1983). An asymmetrical tonic neck reflex rating scale. *American Journal of Occupational Therapy*, 37, 462-465.

Payton, O. E., Hirt, S., & Newton, R. A. (1977). *Neurophysiologic approaches to therapeutic exercise: An anthology.* Philadelphia: F. A. Davis.

Peiper, A. (1963). *Cerebral function in infancy and childhood*. New York: Consultants Bureau.

Rider, B. A. (1972). Tonic neck reflexes. *American Journal of Occupational Therapy*, 26, 132-134.

Shumway-Cook, A., & Woollacott, M. H. (1985). Dynamics of postural control in the child with Down Syndrome. *Physical Therapy*, 65, 1315-1322.

Sieg, K. W., & Shuster, J. J. (1979). Comparison of three positions for evaluating the asymmetrical tonic neck reflex. *American Journal of Occupational Therapy*, 33, 311-316.

Stilwell, J. M., & Heiniger, M. C. (1983). Tilt reactions in sitting in normal and learning disabled children, *Physical & Occupational Therapy in Pediatrics*, 3(4), 43-58.

Stilwell, J. M. (1981). Relationship between development of the body-righting reaction and manual midline crossing behavior in the learning disabled. *American Journal of Occupational Therapy, 35,* 391-398.

Touwen, B. (1984). Primitive reflexes - conceptional or semantic problem? In H. Prechtl (Ed.), *Continuity of neural functions from prenatal to postnatal life. Clinics in developmental medicine No. 94.* Philadelphia: J. B. Lippincott.

Twitchell, T. E. (1969). Early development of the avoiding and grasping reactions. In S. Locke (Ed.), *Modern Neurology* (pp 333-345). Boston, MA: Little Brown & Co.

Weisz, A. (1939). Studies in equilibrium reactions. *Journal of Nervous and Mental Disorders, 88,* 150-162.

Zemke, R. (1980). Incidence of ATNR response in normal preschool children. *Physical & Occupational Therapy in Pediatrics, 1*(2), 31-37.

Zemke, R. (1983). The consistency of the magnitude of the ATNR response in normal preschool children. *Physical & Occupational Therapy in Pediatrics, 3*(3), 57-61.

Zemke, R. (1984). Notes on the measurement of the magnitude of the asymmetrical tonic neck reflex response in normal preschool children. *Journal of Motor Behavior, 16,* 333-336.

Zemke, R. (1985). Application of an ATNR rating scale to normal preschool children. *American Journal of Occupational Therapy, 39,* 178-180.

Sensory Systems/Assessment/Treatment

Ayres, A. J., & Tickle, L. S. (1980). Hyper-responsivity to touch and vestibular stimulation as a predictor of positive response to sensory integration procedures by autistic children. *American Journal of Occupational Therapy,34*,(6) 375-381.

Ayres, A. J. & Mailloux, A. K. (1981). Influence of sensory integration procedures on language development. *American Journal of Occupational Therapy, 35*, 383-390.

Ayres, A. J., & Mailloux, A. K. (1983). Possible pubertal effect on therapeutic gains in an autistic girl. *American Journal of Occupational Therapy, 37*, 535-540.

Azrin, N. H., Kaplan, S. J., & Foxx, R. M. (1973). Eliminating stereotyped self-stimulation of retarded individuals. *American Journal of Mental Defiency, 78*, 241-248.

Bailey, J., & Myerson, L. (1970). Effect of vibratory stimulation on a retardate's self-injurious behavior. *American Journal of Mental Deficiency, 17*, 133-137.

Barton, E. S., & Broughton, S. F. (1980). Stereotyped behaviors in profoundly retarded clients: A review. In E.S. Barton (Ed.), *Behavior Research of Severe Developmental Disabilities, Vol. 1* (pp. 279-306). New York: North Holland Publishing Co.

Bauer, B. A. (1977). Tactile sensitivity: Development of a behavioral responses checklist. *American Journal of Occupational Therapy, 31*, 357-361.

Baumeister, A. A., & Baumeister, A. A. (1978). Suppression of repetitive self-injurious behavior by contingent inhalation of aromatic ammonia. *Journal of Autism and Childhood Schizophrenia, 8*, 71-77.

Bishop, B. (1974). Vibratory stimulation: Part I. Neurophysiology of motor responses evoked by vibratory stimulation. *Physical Therapy, 54*, 1273-1282.

Bishop, B. (1975a). Vibratory stimulation: Part II. Vibratory stimulation as an evaluation tool. *Physical Therapy, 55*, 28-34.

Bishop, B. (1975b). Vibratory stimulation: Part III. Possible applications of vibration in treatment of motor dysfunctions. *Physical Therapy, 55*, 139-143.

Bonadonna, P. (1981). Effects of a vestibular stimulation program on stereo-typic rocking behavior. *American Journal of Occupational Therapy, 35*, 775-781.

Bright, T., Bittick, K., & Fleeman, B. (1981). Reduction of self-injurious behavior using sensory integrative techniques. *American Journal of Occupational Therapy, 35*, 167-172.

Clark, F. A., & Shuer, J. (1978, June). A clarification of sensory integrative therapy and its application to programming with retarded people. *Mental Retardation, 16*(3), .227-232.

Clyse, S. J., & Short, M. A. (1983). Relationship between dynamic balance and postrotary nystagmus in learning disabled children. *Physical & Occupational Therapy in Pediatrics, 3*(3), 25-32.

Colman, R., Frankel, F., Ritvo, E., & Freeman, B. J. (1976). The effects of fluorescent and incandescent illumination upon repetitive behaviors in autistic children. *Journal of Autism and Childhood Schizophrenia, 6*, 157-162.

Condon, W. S. (1975). Multiple response to sound in dysfunctional children. *Journal of Autism and Childhood Schizophrenia, 5*, 37-56.

Demetral, G. D., & Lutzker, J. R. (1980). The parameters of facial screening in treating self-injurious behavior. In E. S. Barton (Ed.) *Behavior Research of Severe Developmental Disabilities 1*, (pp. 261-177). New York: North Holland Publishing Co.

Dichgans, C. L, Schmidt, C. L., & Graf, W. (1973). Visual input improve the speedometer function of the vestibular nuclei in the goldfish. *Experimental Brain Research, 18,* 319-322.

Drabman, R. S., Cordua, Y., Cruz, G., Ross, J., & Lynd, S. (1979). Suppression of chronic drooling in mentally retarded children and adolescents: Effectiveness of a behavioral treatment package. *Behavior Therapy, 10,* 46-56.

Farber, S. (1978). Olfaction in health and disease. *American Journal of Occupational Therapy, 32,* 155-160.

Farber, S., & Huss, A. J. (1974). *Sensorimotor evaluation and treatment procedures.* (2nd ed.). Indianapolis: Indiana University, Indianapolis Medical Center.

Ferster, C. B. (1961). Positive reinforcement and behavioral deficits in autistic children. *Child Development, 32,* 437-456.

Forssberg, H., & Nasher, L. M. (1982). Ontogenetic development of postural control in man: Adaptation to altered support and visual conditions during stance. *Journal of Neuroscience, 2,* 545-552.

Fox, J. (1966). The olfactory system: Implications for the occupational therapist. *American Journal of Ocupational Therapy, 20,* 173-177.

Foxx, R. M. & Azrin, N. H. (1973). Elimination of autistic self-stimulating behavior by overcorrection. *Journal of Applied Behavior Analysis, 6,* 1-14.

Frankel, F., Freeman, B. J., Ritvo, E., & Pardo, R. (1978). The effect of environmental stimulation upon the stereotyped behavior of autistic children. *Journal of Autism and Childhood Schizophrenia, 8,* 389-394.

Freeman, B. J., Frankel, F., & Ritvo, E. R. (1976). The effects of response contingent vestibular stimulation on the behavior of autistic and retarded children. *Journal of Autism and Childhood Schizophrenia, 6,* 353-358.

Griffin, J. (1974). Use of proprioceptive stimuli in therapeutic exercise. *Physical Therapy, 54,* 1072-1079.

Haron, M., & Henderson, A. (1985). Active and passive touch in developmentally dyspraxic and normal boys. *Occupational Therapy Journal of Research, 5,* 101-112.

Hirama, H. (1988). *Self-injurious behavior: A somatosensory treatment approach.* Baltimore, MD:Chess Publications.

Horner, R. D., & Barton, E. S. (1980). Operant techniques in the analysis and modification of self-injurious behavior: A review. In E. S. Barton . (Ed.),*Behavior Research of Severe Developmental Disabilities I,* (pp. 123-130). New York: North Holland Publishing Co.

Hung, D. W. (1978). Using self-stimulation as reinforcement in autistic children. *Journal of Autism and Childhood Schizophrenia, 8,* 355-365.

Hutt, C., & Dunsted, C. (1966). The biological significance of gaze aversion with particular reference to the syndrome of infantile autism. *Behavioral Science, 2,* 346-356.

Jones, F. H. Simmons, J. Q., & Frankel, F. (1974). An extinction procedure for eliminating self-destructive behavior in a 9 year old girl. *Journal of Autism and Childhood Schizophrenia, 4,* 241-248.

Kantner, R. M., Kantner, B., & Clark, D. L. (1982). Vestibular stimulation effect on language development in mentally retarded children. *American Journal of Occupational Therapy, 36,* 36-41.

Katz, R. C., & Lutzker, J. R. (1980). A comparison of three methods for training timeout. In E.S. Barton. (Ed.). *Behavior Research of Severe Development Disabilities,* I, (pp.123-130). New York: North Holland Publishing Co.

Kinnealey, M. (1973). Aversive and non-aversive responses to sensory stimulation in mentally retarded children. *American Journal of Occupational Therapy, 27,* 464-471.

Larson, K. A. (1982). The sensory history of developmentally delayed children with and without tactile defensiveness. *American Journal of Occupational Therapy, 36,* 590-596.

Lemke, H. (1974). Self-abusive behavior in the mentally retarded. *American Journal of Occupational Therapy, 28,* 94-98.

Lovaas, O.I., & Simmons, J. Q. (1969). Manipulation of self-destruction in three retarded children. *Journal of Applied Behavior Analysis, 2,* 143-147.

Magrun, W. M., Ottenbacher, K., McCue, S., & Keefe, R. (1981). Effects of vestibular stimulation on spontaneous use of verbal language in developmentally delayed children. *American Journal of Occupational Therapy, 35,* 101-104.

McKibbin, E. (1973). The effect of additional tactile stimulation in a perceptual-motor treatment program for school children. *American Journal of Occupational Therapy, 27,* 191-197.

Melzack, R., Konrad, K., & Dubrovsky, B. (1969). Prolonged changes in CNS activity produced by somatic and reticular stimulation. *Experimental Neurology, 25,* 416-428.

Montagu A. (1977). *Touching: The human significance of the skin.* New York: Harper & Row.

Montgomery, P. C. (1985). Sensory information and geographical orientation in healthy subjects. *Physical Therapy, 65,* 1471-1477.

Montgomery, P. C., & Capps, M. J. (1980). Effect of arousal on the nystagmus response of normal children. *Physical & Occupational Therapy in Pediatrics, 1*(2), 17-29.

Montgomery, P. C., & Gauger, J. (1978). Sensory dysfunction in children who toe-walk. *Physical Therapy, 58,* 1195-1204.

Montgomery, P. C., & Rodel, D. M. (1982). Effect of state on nystagmus duration on the Southern California Postrotary Nystagmus Test. *American Journal of Occupational Therapy, 36,* 177-182.

Nasher, L. M., Black, F. O., & Wall, C. (1982). Adaptation to altered support and visual conditions during stance: Patients with vestibular deficits. *Journal of Neuroscience, 2,* 536-544.

Nasher, L. M., Shumway-Cook, A., & Marin, O. (1983). Stance posture control in select groups of children with cerebral palsy: Deficits in sensory organization and muscular coordination. *Experimental Brain Research, 49,* 393-409.

Noback, C., & Demarest, R. (1981). *The Human Nervous System.* New York: McGraw-Hill.

Nunes, D. L., Murphy, R. J., & Doughty, N. R. (1980). An interlocking progressive-ratio procedure for determining the reinforcer preferences of multhandicapped children. In E. S. Barton (Ed.) *Behavior Research of Severe Developmental Disabilities,* I, (pp. 161-174). New York: North Holland Publishing Co.

Ornitz, E. M. (1970). Vestibular dysfunction in schizophrenia and childhood autism. *Comprehensive Psychiatry, 2,* 159-173.

Ornitz, E. M. (1974). The modulation of sensory input and motor output in autistic children. *Journal of Autism and Childhood Schizophrenia, 4,* 197-216.

Ornitz, E. M., Brown, M. B., Mason, A., & Putnam, N. H. (1974). Effect of visual input on vestibular nystagmus in autistic children. *Archives of General Psychiatry, 32,* 369-375.

Ornitz, E. M., Forsythe, A. B., & de la Pena, A. (1973). The effect of vestibular and auditory stimulation in the rapid eye movement of REM sleep in normal and autistic children. *Archives of General Psychiatry, 29,* 786-791.

Ottenbacher, K.J. (1982). Patterns of postrotary nystagmus in three learning-disabled children. *American Journal of Occupational Therapy, 36,* 657-663.

Ottenbacher, K. J. (1982). Sensory integration therapy: Affect or effect. *American Journal of Occupational Therapy, 36,* 571-578.

Ottenbacher, K. J., & Short, M. A. (Eds.). (1985). Vestibular processing dysfunction in children. *Physical & Occupational Therapy in Pediatrics, 5*(2/3).

Peiper, A. (1963). *Cerebral function in infancy and childhood.* New York: Consultants Bureau November (1975).

Prescott, J. W. Body pleasure and the origins of violence. *Bulletin of Atomic Science,* 10-20.

Pribram, K. H., & McGuinness, D. (1975). Arousal, activation, and efforts in the control of attention. *Psychological Review, 32,* 116-149.

Purpura, D. P. (1974). Dendritic spine dysgenesis and mental retardation. *Science, 186,* 1126-1128.

deQuiros, J. B. (1976). Diagnosis of vestibular disorders in the learning disabled. *Journal of Learning Disabilities, 9,* 50-58.

Resman, M. H. (1981). Effect of sensory stimulation on eye contact in a profoundly retarded adult. *American Journal of Occupational* Therapy, *35,* 31-35.

Richmond, G., & Bell, J. C. (1983). Analysis of a treatment package to reduce a hand-mouthing stereotype. *Behavior Therapy, 14,* 576-581.

Rincover, A. (1978). Sensory extinction: A procedure for eliminating self-stimulatory behavior in developmentally disabled children. *Journal of Abnormal Child Psychology, 6,* 299-310.

Rincover, A., Cook, R., Peoples, A., & Packard, D. (1979). Sensory extinction and sensory reinforcement principles for programming multiple and adative behavior changes. *Journal of Applied Behavior Analysis, 12,* 221-233.

Ritvo, E., & Ornitz, E. M. (1968). Frequency of repetitive behaviors in early infantile autism and its variants. *Archives of Genetic Psychology, 19,* 341-347.

Rosenweig, M. R. (1976). Effects of environment on brain and behavior in animals. In E. Schopler & R. J. Reichler (Eds.), *Psychopathology and child development* (pp. 33-50). New York: Plenum Press.

Ross, E. F. (1984). Review and critique of research on the use of tactile and kinesthetic stimulation with premature infants. *Physical & Occupational Therapy in Pediatrics, 4*(1), 35-49.

Rotegal, M. (1982). Vestibular and neostriatal contributions to spatial orientation. In *Spatial abilities: Development and physiological foundations,* (pp. 361-382). New York: Academic Press.

Royeen, C. B. (1985a). Domain specifications of the construct tactile defensiveness. *American Journal of Occupational Therapy, 39,* 596-599.

Royeen, C. B. (1985b). The development of a touch scale for measuring tactile defensiveness in children. *American Journal of Occupational Therapy, 40,* 414-419.

Sallustro, F., & Atwell, C. W. (1978). Body rocking, head banging, and head rolling in normal children. *Journal of Pediatrics, 93,*(4) 704-708.

Sarnet, H. B., & Netsky, M. G. (1979). *Evaluation of the nervous system.* New York: Oxford Press.

Schopler, E. (1965). Early infantile autism and receptor processes. *Archives of General Psychiatry, 13,* 327-335

Short, M. A., Watson, P. J., Ottenbacher, K., & Rogers, C. (1983). Vestibular-proprioceptive functions in 4 year olds: Normative and regression analyses. *American Journal of Occupational Therapy, 37,* 103-109.

Storey, K. Bates, P., McGhee, N., & Dycus, S. (1984). Reducing the self-stimulatory behavior of a profoundly retarded female through sensory awareness training. *American Journal of Occupational Therapy, 38,* 510-516.

Walsh, R. N., & Cummins, R. A. (1976). Neural responses to therapeutic environments. In R. N. Walsh & W. T. Greenbough, (Eds.) *Environment as therapy for brain dysfunctions.*(pp. 171-200). New York: Plenum Press.

Weeks, Z. R. (1979a). Effects of vestibular system on human development. Part I. Overview of function and effects of stimulation, *American Journal of Occupational Therapy, 33,* 376-381.

Weeks, Z. R. (1979). Part 2. Effects of vestibular system stimulation on mentally retarded, emotionally disturbed, and learning disabled individuals. *American Journal of Occupational Therapy, 33,* 450-457.

Zuckerman, M. (1979). *Sensation seeking: Beyond the optimal level of arousal.* Hillsdale, N. J.: Lawrence Erlbaum Associates.

Appendix F

Treatment/Intervention/Programming

Anderson, J. (1986). Sensory intervention with the preterm infant in the neonatal intensive care unit. *American Journal of Occupational Therapy, 40,* 19-26.

Arnold, E., Clark, D., Sachs, L., Jakim, S., & Smithies, C. (1985). Vestibular and visual rotational stimulation as treatment for attention deficit and hyperactivity. *American Journal of Occupational Therapy, 39,* 84-91.

Ayres, A. J. (1972). Improving academic scores through sensory integration. *Journal of Learning Disabilities, 5,* 338-342.

Ayres, A. J. (1976). *The effect of sensory integrative therapy on learning disabled children: The final report of a research project.* Pasadena, CA: The Center for the study of Sensory Integrative Dysfunction.

Ayres, A. J. (1977). Effect of sensory integrative therapy on the coordination of children with choreoathetoid movements. *American Journal of Occupational Therapy, 31,* 291-293.

Ayres, A. J. (1978). Learning disabilities and the vestibular system. *Journal of Learning Disabilites, 11,* 30-41.

Ayres, A. J., Mailloux, Z. (1981). Influence of sensory integration procedures on language development. *American Journal of Occupational Therapy, 35,* 383-390.

Bailey, D. M. (1978). The effects of vestibular stimulation on verbalizations in chronic schizophrenics. *American Journal of Occupational Therapy, 37,* 445-450.

Bauer, B. A. (1977). Tactile sensitive behavior in hyperactive and non-hyperactive children. *American Journal of Occupational Therapy, 31,* 447-453.

Bissell, J., Fisher, J., Owens, C., & Polcyn, P. (1988). *Handbook of sensorimotor activities.* Torrence, CA: Sensory Integration International.

Bhatara, V., Clark, D. L., & Arnold, L. E. (1978). Behavioral and nystagmus response of a hyperactive child to vestibular stimulation. *American Journal of Occupational Therapy, 32,* 311-316.

Bobath, B. (1963). Treatment principles and planning in cerebral palsy. *Physiotherapy, 49,* 122-124.

Boehme, R. (1988). *Improving upper body control: An approach to assessment and treatment.* Tucson, AZ: Therapy Skill Builders.

Brody, F. J., Thomas, J. A., Brody, O. R., & Kucherway, D. A. (1977). Comparisons of sensory integration and operant methods for production of vocalization in profoundly retarded adults. *Perceptual and Motor Skills, 44,* 1283-1296.

Campbell, S. (1974). Facilitation of cognitive and motor development in infants with central nervous system dysfunction. *Physical Therapy, 54* (4), 346-353.

Campbell, S., & Wilson, J. (1976). Planning infant learning programs. *Physical Therapy, 56,* 1347-1357.

Chee, F. K. W., Kreutzberg, J. R., & Clark, D. L. (1978). Semicircular canal stimulation in cerebral palsied children. *Physical Therapy, 58,* 1221-1227.

Clark, D. L., Kreutzberg, J. R. & Chee, F. (1977). Vestibular-stimulation influence on motor development in infants, *Science, 196,* 1228-1229.

Clark, F. A., Miller, L. R., Thomas, J. A., Kucherawy, D. A., & Azen, S. P. (1978). A comparison of operant and sensory integrative methods on vocalization and other developmental parameters in profoundly retarded adults. *American Journal of Occupational Therapy, 32,* 86-92.

Conner, F., Williams, G., & Siepp, J. (1978). *Program guide for infants and toddlers with neuromotor and other developmental disabilities.* New York: Teachers College Press.

Connolly, B. H., Margon, S., & Russell, F. F. (1984). Evaluation of children with Down Syndrome who participated in an early intervention program. *Physical Therapy, 64,* 1515-1519.

Connolly, B. H., & Montgomery, P. C. (1987). *Therapeutic exercise in developmental disabilities.* Chattanooga, TN: Chattanooga Publishing.

Crowe, T. (1981). Father involvement in early intervention programs. *Physical & Occupational Therapy in Pediatrics, 1*(3), 35-46.

Edgar, C. L., Ball, T. S., McIntyre, R. B., & Shotwell, A. M. (1969). Effects of sensory-motor training on adaptive behavior. *American Journal of Occupational Therapy, 73,* 713-720.

Erhardt, R. (1982). *Developmental hand dysfunction.* Laurel, MD: RAMSCO Publishing Co.

Esenther, S. E. (1984). Developmental coaching of the Down Syndrome infant. *American Journal of Occupational Therapy, 38,* 440-445.

Fiebert, I. M. (1979). Vestibular stimulation to improve ambulation after a cerebral vascular accident. *Physical Therapy, 4,* 423-426.

Finnie, N. (1975). *Handling the young cerebral palsied child at home.* New York: E. P. Dutton & Company.

Freeman, B. J., Frankel, F., & Ritvo, E. D. (1976). The effect of response contingent vestibular stimulation on the behavior of autistic and retarded children. *Journal of Autism and Childhood Schizophrenia, 6,* 353-358.

Gregg, C., Haffner, M., & Korner, A. (1976). The relative efficacy of vestibular-proprioceptive stimulation and the upright position in enhancing visual pursuit in neonates. *Child Development, 47,* 309-314.

Griffin, J. (1974). Use of proprioceptive stimuli in therapeutic exercise. *Physical Therapy, 54,* 1072-1079.

Grimwood, L. M., & Rutherford, E. M. (1980). Sensory integration therapy as an intervention procedure with grade one "at risk" readers - a three year study. *Exceptional Child, 27,* 52-61.

Huff, D.M, & Harris, S. C. (1987). Using sensorimotor integrative treatment with mentally retarded adults. *American Journal of Occupational Therapy, 41,* 227-231.

Illingworth, R. S. (1966). The diagnosis of cerebral palsy in the first year of life. *Developmental Medicine and Child Neurology, 8,* 178-194.

Jenkins, J. R., Sells, C., Brady, D., Down, J., Moore, B., Carman, P., & Holm, R. (1982). Effects of developmental therapy on motor impaired children, *Occupational & Physical Therapy in Pediatrics, 2*(4)19-28.

Kantner, R., Clark, D., Allen, L., & Chase, M. (1976). Effects of vestibular stimulation on nystagmus response and motor performance in the developmentally delayed infant. *Physical Therapy, 56,*.414-421.

Kantner, R., Kantner, B., & Clark, D. (1982). Vestibular stimulation effect on language development in mentally retarded children. *American Journal of Ocupational Therapy, 36,* 36-41.

Kearsley, R., & Sigel, I. (Eds.). (1979). *Infant at risk: Assessment of cognitive functioning.* Hillsdale, New Jersey: Lawrence Erlbaum Associates, Inc.

Kimball, J. G. (1986). Prediction of Methylophenidate (Ritalin) responsiveness through sensory integrative testing, *American Journal of Occupational Therapy, 40,* 241-248.

King, L. J. (1974). A sensory integration approach to schizophrenia. *American Journal of Occupational Therapy, 28,* 529-536.

Kong, E. (1966). Very early treatment of cerebral palsy. *Developmental Medicine and Child Neurology, 8,* 198-202

Kopp, B. (1974). Application of Piagetian theory: Sensory-motor development. *American Journal of Occupational Therapy, 28,* 217-219.

Korner, A. F. (1973). Early stimulation and maternal care as related to infant capabilities and individual differences. *Early Child Development and Care, 2,* 307-327.

Korner, A. F., & Grobstein, R. (1966). Visual alertness as related to soothing in neonates: Implications for maternal stimulation and early deprivation. *Child Development, 37*, 867-876.

Korner, A. F., Kraemer, H., Haffner, M., & Cosper, L.(1975). Effects of waterbed floatation on premature infants: A pilot study. *Pediatrics, 56*, 361-367.

Korner, A. F., Gregg, C., & Hoffner, M. (1976). The relative efficacy of vestibular-proprioceptive stimulation and the upright position in enhancing visual pursuit in neonates. *Child Development, 47*, 309-314.

Kranser, L., & Pierpont, M. (1976). Rocking waterbeds and auditory stimulation to enhance growth of preterm infants. *Journal of Pediatrics, 88*, 297-299.

Levine, S., & Kliebhan, L. (1981). Communication between physician and physical and occupational therapists: A neurodevelopmentally-based prescription. *Pediatrics, 68*, 208-214.

MacLean, W. E., & Baumeister, A. A. (1982). Effects of vestibular stimulation on motor development and stereotyped behavior of developmentally delayed children. *Journal of Abnormal Child Psychology, 10*, 229-245.

Miller, T. G. (1975). Sensorimotor integration: An interdisciplinary approach. *Physical Therapy, 55*, 501-504.

Montgomery, P. & Richter, E. (1977). Effect of sensory integrative therapy on the neuromotor development of retarded children. *Physical Therapy, 57*, 799-806.

Montgomery, P. C. & Richter, E. (2nd Ed., 1989). *Sensorimotor integration for developmentaly disabled children: A handbook*. Los Angeles: Western Psychological Services.

Nelson, D. (1984). *Children with autism and other pervasive disorders of development and behavior: Therapy through activities*. Thorofare, NJ: Charles B. Slack.

Ottenbacher, K. J. (1982). Sensory integration therapy: Affect or effect. *American Journal of Occupational Therapy, 36*, 571-578.

Ottenbacher, K. J. (1983a). Development and treatment of oral-motor dysfunction: A review of clinical research, *Occupational & Physical Therapy in Pediatrics, 3*(92), 1-13.

Ottenbacher, K. (1983b). Transdisciplinary service delivery in school environments: Some limitations. *Occupational & Physical Therapy in Pediatrics, 3*(4), 9-16.

Ottenbacher, K. J., Biocca, Z., DeCremer, G., Gevelinger, M., Jedlovec, K.B., & Johnson, M. B. (1986). Quantitative analysis of the effectiveness of pediatric therapy: Emphasis on the neurodevelopmental approach. *Physical Therapy, 66*, 1095-1101.

Ottenbacher, K.J., Short, M.A., & Watson, P.J. (1979). Nystagmus duration changes of learning disabled children during sensory integrative therapy. *American Journal of Occupational Therapy, 36*, 571-578.

Ottenbacher, K. J., Short, M. A., & Watson, P. J. (1981). The effects of a clinically applied program of vestibular stimulation on the neuromotor performance of children with severe developmental disability. *Physical & Occupational Therapy in Pediatrics, 1*(1), 1-11.

Pehoski, C. (Ed.). (1986). *Play: A skill for life*. Rockville, MD: American Occupational Therapy Association.

Pierson, P., & Williams, C. (Eds.). (1976). *Physical therapy services in the developmental disabilities*. Springfield, IL: Charles C. Thomas.

Powell, L. F. (1974). The effect of extra stimulation and maternal involvement on the development of low birthweight infants and on maternal behavior. *Child Development, 45*, 106-113.

deQuiros, J. (1976). Diagnosis of vestibular disorders in the learning disabled. *Journal of Learning Disabilities, 9*(1), 50-58.

Redditi, J. S. (1983). Occupational and physical therapy treatment components for infant intervention programs. *Physical & Occupational Therapy in Pediatrics, 3*(3), 33-44.

Reilly, C., Nelson, D., & Bundy, A. (1983). Sensorimotor vs. fine motor activities in eliciting vocalizations in autistic children. *Occupational Therapy Journal of Research, 3*, 199-212.

Resnick, R., & Zemke, R. (1980). Piaget, pre-school and pediatric practice, *Occupational & Physical Therapy in Pediatrics, 1*(1), 3-9.

Rider, B. A. (1978). Sensorimotor treatment of chronic schizophrenics. *American Journal of Occupational Therapy, 32,* 451-455.

Ross, E. F. (1984). Review and critique of research on the use of tactile and kinesthetic stimulation with premature infants. *Occupational & Physical Therapy in Pediatrics, 4,*(1) 35-49.

Scherzer, A. L. & Tscharnuter, I. (1982). *Early diagnosis and therapy in cerebral palsy.* New York: Marcel Dekker, Inc.

Solkoff, N., Yaffe, S., Weintraub, D., & Blase, B. (1969). Effects of handling on the subsequent development of premature infants. *Developmental Medicine, 1,* 765-768.

Tjossem, T. (Ed.). (1976). *Intervention strategies for high risk infants and young children.* Baltimore: University Park Press.

SPA Criteria

Client rolls approximately twelve feet in a straight line from one designated point to another (place masking tape line on carpet or mat). Client rolls back in the opposite direction. Encourage client to roll slowly. Demonstrate if necessary.

A-1. ROLLS BOTH DIRECTIONS
Poor: Client rolls to one side only.

Inadequate: Client tends to roll to one direction, but will roll both directions when encouraged. (Check to which side client does *not* roll spontaneously.)

Optimal: Client rolls to *both* sides easily and spontaneously.

A-2. MOTOR PLANNING
Poor: Cannot roll from one point to another; may roll in circular pattern.

Inadequate: Has some difficulty rolling in a straight line, but can correct himself to arrive at correct point.

Optimal: Rolls easily in a straight line in both directions (Fig. 1, 2).

Note: If asymmetry in response, check to which side (body space) client has *more* difficulty motor planning.

A-3. BODY RIGHTING
Poor: Log rolls, no segmentation of hip, trunk, or shoulders (Fig. 1, 2).

Inadequate: Log rolls, but occasionally uses segmental movement or log rolls to only one side (Fig. 5).

Optimal: Smooth segmental roll in both directions with hip or shoulder leading.

Note: If asymmetry in response, check side to which client rolls *not* using body righting.

A-4. HEAD RIGHTING
Poor: As client rolls, head touches floor occasionally or cannot be lifted off surface at all (Fig. 2, 3, 4).

Inadequate: Client lifts head up, but occasionally drops it without touching floor (Fig. 1, 2, 5).

Optimal: Head rights in all positions and does not touch floor.
Evaluate in prone, supine, and lateral positions during roll.

Scoring Instructions: Prone (a) response is placed in Antigravity Extension box (Fig. 2, 3); Supine (b) (Fig. 1, 4) placed in Antigravity Flexion box; lowest score recorded is placed in the other open boxes on the Profile.

A-5. ASYMMETRICAL TONIC NECK PATTERN (ATNR)
Poor: Client uses ATNR to roll by turning face to elicit arm extension and build up momentum for rolling. [Note: Check direction face is turned if ATNR response occurs] (Fig. 5).

Inadequate: Client occasionally uses ATNR to roll.

Optimal: Client rotates with opposite shoulder (if using ATNR, same arm will lead). Evaluate in both directions.

A-6. ANTIGRAVITY FLEXION
Poor: Client routinely assumes *hyperextended* position of neck and/or trunk when supine (Fig. 4).

Inadequate: Client occasionally assumes *hyperextended* position when supine.

Optimal: Client assumes extended position of trunk momentarily when supine.

A-7. ANTIGRAVITY EXTENSION
Poor: Client assumes flexed posture when prone [Note whether hips, knees and/or arms are flexed] (Fig. 2, 3).

Inadequate: Mild flexion is evident when in prone position.

Optimal: Client does not flex when in prone position.

A-8. BECOMES DIZZY (VESTIBULAR)
Poor: Client reports or displays dizziness/nausea or becomes disoriented and cannot complete task.

Inadequate: Client reports dizziness/nausea or becomes disoriented but can complete task with some difficulty.

Optimal: Client reports mild dizziness but does not become disoriented and completes task easily.

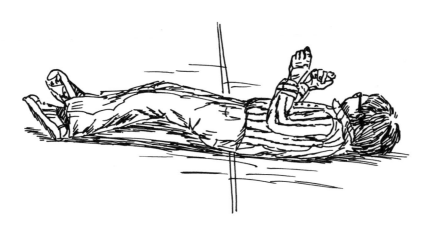

Figure 1
Task: Rolling
Scoring
A-3.   Body Righting: Score (1), no segmentation of hip, trunk, or shoulders
A-4.   Head Righting: Score (2), occasionally drops head without touching floor

Comment: Slow rolling prevents log rolling as a result of momentum and allows the examiner to observe the trunk more carefully.

To evaluate trunk rotation, draw an imaginary line from hip to shoulder. If the line is diagonal, trunk segmentation is occurring. The child in this illustration has a straight line and is demonstrating trunk rigidity.

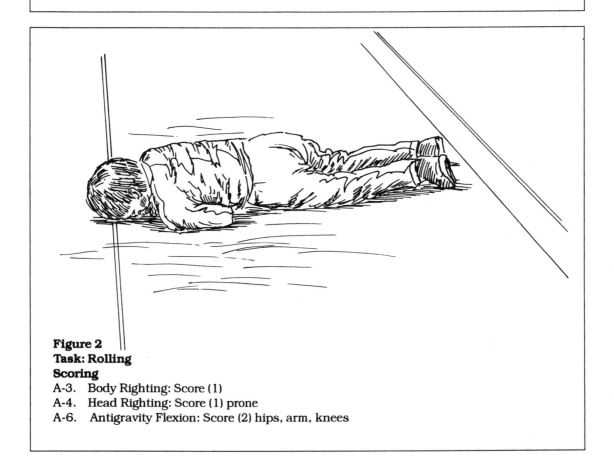

Figure 2
Task: Rolling
Scoring
A-3.   Body Righting: Score (1)
A-4.   Head Righting: Score (1) prone
A-6.   Antigravity Flexion: Score (2) hips, arm, knees

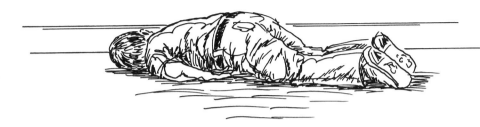

Figure 3
Task: Rolling
Scoring
A-4.   Head Righting: Score (1) head touches floor (prone)
A-7.   Antigravity Extension: Score (1) flexed posture when prone (check hips, knees, arms)

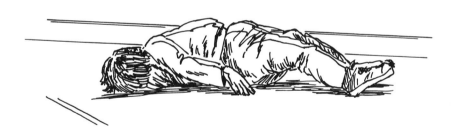

Figure 4
Task: Rolling
Scoring
A-2.   Motor Planning: Score (1) cannot roll from one point to another
A-3.   Body Righting: Score (1) log rolls (although trunk is arched, shoulder and hip are still aligned)
A-4.   Head Righting: Score (1) cannot lift off surface (supine)
A-6.   Antigravity Flexion: Score (1) hyperextended position

Comment: Notice the excessive extension of the trunk used to initiate roll.

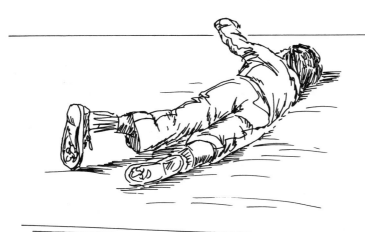

Figure 5
Task: Rolling
Scoring
A-2. Motor Planning: Score (1) cannot roll from one point to another
A-3. Body Righting: Score (3) some segmental movement while initiating roll, then log rolls
A-4. Head Righting: Score (2) drops head without touching floor
A-5. Asymmetrical Tonic Neck: Score (1) uses ATNR to roll (check left)

Comment: This child illustrates the use of the asymmetrical tonic neck pattern to initiate rotation.

Client crawls on stomach approximately fifteen feet on tile or other nonresistive surface. Ask client to crawl as fast as he can on an "S" curved line (use masking tape for line). Demonstrate if necessary using all four extremities.

B-1. MOTOR PLANNING
Poor: Cannot crawl from one point to another along curved line (Fig. 6, 7, 8).
Inadequate: Has difficulty crawling along curved line, but can correct position and end up at designated point.
Optimal: Can crawl easily on curved line.

B-2. HAND POSITION
Poor: Patterns a) pulls with forearms not hands, b) hands fisted, c) fingertips only, d) palms only used primarily (Fig. 9).
Inadequate: Patterns a,b,c, and d used intermittently with pattern e) uses whole hand to pull (Fig. 6, 7, 11, 12).
Optimal: Pattern e (Fig. 8, 10).
Note position of hands as client is crawling.

B-3. EXTREMITY LAG
Poor: Consistently neglects one extremity (Fig. 8, 9).
Note which extremity is neglected.
Inadequate: Occasionally neglects one extremity.
Optimal: Uses all four extremities.

B-4. PROPULSION
Poor: Either feet or knees are used for pushing or both legs lag (Fig. 6, 7, 10).
Inadequate: Occasionally feet and knees push together (Fig. 11, 12).
Optimal: Feet and knees push together consistently (Fig. 9).

B-5. ANTI-GRAVITY EXTENSION
Poor: Persistently maintains significant hip flexion in prone on one or both sides (Fig. 9, 11, 12).
Inadequate: Persistently maintains slight hip flexion on one or both sides in prone, or occasionally maintains significant hip flexion on one or both sides.
Optimal: Hips rotate and fully extend in prone position.

B-6. PRONE HEAD RIGHTING
Poor: Cannot lift chin off floor (Fig. 11).
Inadequate: Looks down at floor; occasionally drops chin to floor; cannot maintain neck extension (Fig. 6).
Optimal: Maintains neck extension, face rights to vertical during crawling (Fig. 7, 8, 9).

B-7. UPPER TRUNK EXTENSION
Poor: Client crawls with upper trunk flat on floor; a very labored crawl or substitutes neck hyperextension (Fig. 7, 11, 12).
Inadequate: Client occasionally uses upper trunk extension off floor (Fig. 6, 8, 10).
Optimal: Client uses upper trunk extension to facilitate a crawling pattern so that forearm weight-bearing is perpendicular to the shoulder joint (Fig. 9).

B-8. LATERAL TRUNK MOVEMENT
Poor: Trunk remains rigid, little lateral movement is evident (Fig. 7, 10).
Inadequate: Lateral movement occasionally or to one side only (Fig. 6, 9, 11, 12).
Optimal: Lateral trunk movement occurs alternately to both sides during crawling.

B-9. CRAWLING PATTERN
Note type of pattern: If client moves head side to side in homolateral pattern, assess influence of ATNR (Fig. 6); if head moves up and down in homologous pattern, assess influence of STNR (Fig. 7, 8).
Poor: Patterns a) homolateral (Fig. 10, 11) or b) homologous used primarily (Fig. 7, 8).
Inadequate: Patterns a or b used intermittently with c) reciprocal.
Optimal: Pattern c.
Scoring Instruction: Homolateral/ATNR (a) under ATNR; Homologous/STNR (b) under STNR; place lowest score in other open boxes on Profile.

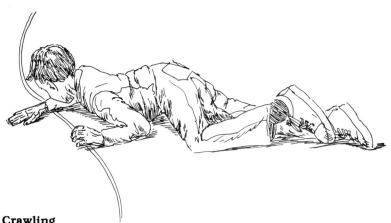

Figure 6
Task: Belly Crawling
Scoring
B-1. Motor Planning: Score (1) cannot crawl from one point to another along curved line
B-2. Hand Position: Score (3) pulls with forearms and hands
B-4. Propulsion: Score (1) uses knees to push
B-6. Prone Head Righting: Score (3) looks down at floor as crawls
B-7. Upper Trunk Extension: Score (2) occasionally uses upper trunk extension off floor
B-8. Lateral Trunk Movement: Score (2) lateral movement occasionally noted

Comment: Head positioning indicates the influence of asymetrical tonic neck patterning which leads to a homolateral crawling pattern. Notice the poor extensor tone in the neck and upper trunk which places the center of gravity in the thorax region.

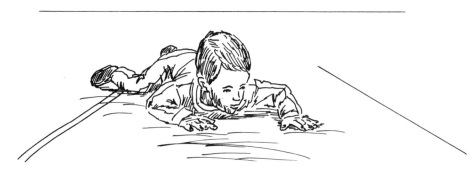

Figure 7
Task: Belly Crawling
Scoring
B-1. Motor Planning: Score (1) cannot crawl along curved line
B-6. Prone Head Righting: Score (2) cannot maintain neck extension
B-7. Upper Trunk Extension: Score (1) upper trunk flat on floor
B-8. Lateral Trunk Movement: Score (1) trunk rigid; little lateral movement noted
B-9. Crawling Pattern: Score (2) primarily homologous with some reciprocation of upper extremities noted

Comment: Although this child is achieving some headrighting, he is clearly not getting upper trunk extension for weight bearing on elbows. Position of the arms in relation to the shoulder is developmentally about 2 months. The symmetrical position of the arms indicate the use of a homologous-type crawling pattern.

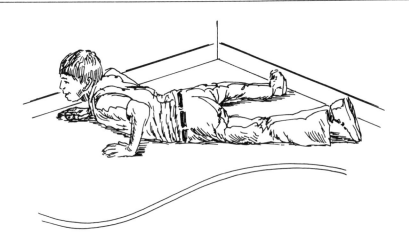

Figure 8
Task: Belly Crawling
Scoring
B-1. Motor Planning: Score (1) cannot crawl along curved line
B-2. Hand Position: Score (5)
B-3. Extremity Lag: Score (1) consistently neglects one extremity (check left)
B-7. Upper Trunk Extension: Score (3) occasionally uses upper trunk extension
B-9. Crawling Pattern: Score (1) homolateral used intermittently with homologous

Comment: Hyperextension of the neck indicates poor balance between neck flexors, and extensors. Again, trunk extension and weight bearing on elbows is very poor quality. This child does not seem to be getting a good push with his feet.

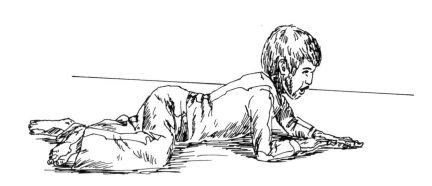

Figure 9
Task: Belly Crawling
Scoring
B-2. Hand Position: Score (1) uses palms and forearms
B-3. Extremity Lag: Score (1) neglects left leg (check lt __ , circle LE)
B-4. Propulsion: Score (5)
B-5. Anti-Gravity Extension: Score (1) maintains hip flexion
B-7. Upper-Trunk Extension: Score (4)
B-8. Lateral Trunk Movement: Score (2) lateral movement occasionally, usually to one side

Comment: Excessive hip flexion and unilateral leg use is a common pattern. Children with poor sensorimotor integration will often tend to use one side of their body for the majority of their weight bearing and the other side for mobility patterns.

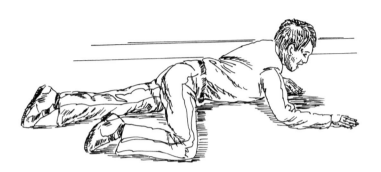

Figure 10
Task: Belly Crawling
Scoring
B-7.   Upper-Trunk Extension: Score (3)
B-8.   Lateral Trunk Movement: Score (1)
B-9.   Crawling Pattern: Score (1) homolateral

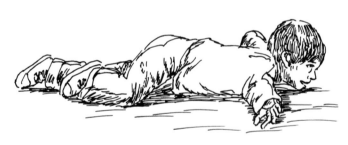

Figure 11
Task: Belly Crawling
Scoring
B-2   Hand Position: Score (1) intermittent pattern
B-4.   Propulsion: Score (3)
B-5.   Anti-Gravity Extension: Score (1) maintains hip flexion
B-6.   Prone Head Righting: Score (1) cannot lift child off floor
B-7.   Upper Trunk Extension: Score (1) upper trunk flat on floor
B-8.   Lateral Trunk Movement: Score (2) lateral movement occasionally noted
B-9.   Crawling Pattern: a. Homolateral, score (1)

Comment: Notice that this child's weight is coming down on the neck and chin, a typical pattern in the newborn. (The child in Fig. 11 and 12 is the same child.)

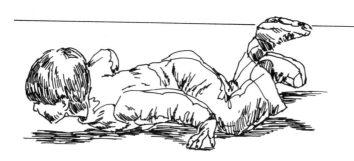

Figure 12
Task: Belly Crawling
Scoring:

B-2   Hand Position: Score (3) intermittent patterns
B-4. Propulsion: Score (3) uses knees for pushing, occasionally feet assist (see Fig. 11)
B-5. Anti-Gravity Extension: Score (1) persistently maintains significant hip flexion in prone on both sides
B-6. Prone Head Righting: Score (2) cannot maintain neck extension
B-7. Upper Trunk Extension: Score (1) upper trunk flat on floor, labored crawl

Comment: As the child attempts to weight shift by lifting his head, he gets increased flexor tonus in his lower extremities and uses capitol extension of the neck. Weight is shifted only as far back as the upper trunk.

Swing suspended ball horizontally at eye level as the client maintains an all-fours position and observe eye tracking. Then have client bat ball horizontally several times (test bilaterally). Demonstrate if necessary.

C-1. MAINTAINS FOUR-POINT POSITION
Poor: Cannot maintain quadruped position—sits back on heels, one or both arms cannot support weight (Fig. 14).
Inadequate: Maintains quadruped position momentarily.
Optimal: Able to support trunk in quadruped position throughout test (Fig. 13).

C-2. EYE TRACKING
Poor: Cannot visually follow swinging ball.
Inadequate: Has difficulty visually tracking ball.
Optimal: Visually follows swinging ball with ease.

C-3. VISUAL AVOIDING REACTION
Poor: Continuously looks away or closes eyes when presented with the ball.
Inadequate: Occasionally focuses on ball.
Optimal: Focuses easily and continuously on ball.

C-4. CROSSES MIDLINE VISUALLY
Poor: Eyes do not cross vertical midline of body; client may tilt head or move body to avoid crossing midline.
Inadequate: Eyes jerk at midline, but client is able to cross midline visually.
Optimal: Eyes cross midline in a smooth continuous movement.

C-5. CROSSES MIDLINE MOTORICALLY
Poor: Hitting arm does not cross vertical midline of body; client may move body or hit ball from midline out to avoid crossing midline (Fig. 15, 16, 17).
Inadequate: Hitting arm crosses midline occasionally, but not consistently.
Optimal: Hitting arm crosses midline consistently and trunk rotation is present.
Note: Check which arm does not cross midline normally.

C-6. HEAD RIGHTING
Poor: Head remains in a tilted or flexed position.
Inadequate: Head occasionally tilts or drops down (Fig. 17).
Optimal: Head remains in good alignment with body and face is vertical to floor (Fig. 16).

C-7. SYMMETRICAL TONIC NECK
Poor: Supporting arm(s) flexes if head drops down; client has tendency to sit back on heels; client can only hit swinging ball if head is hyperextended (Fig. 14, 15).
Inadequate: Client occasionally flexes and extends support arm(s) as head moves up and down; occasionally sits back on heels (Fig. 17).
Optimal: Client maintains extension in support arm(s) regardless of head position.

C-8. HAND POSITION OF SUPPORT ARMS
Poor: a) fisted (Fig. 15), b) fingertips only (Fig. 16), or c) palms only (Fig. 13).
Inadequate: Pattern a,b, or c used intermittently with d) whole hand flat.
Optimal: Pattern d (Fig. 17).
Note: If asymmetry is observed, check left or right and score the poorest response on Profile.

C-9. HAND POSITION OF HITTING ARM
Poor: a) fisted, b) fingertips only, or c) palms only.
Inadequate: Patterns a, b, or c used intermittently with d) whole hand.
Optimal: Pattern d.
Note: If asymmetry is observed, check left or right and score the poorest response on Profile.

C-10. MAINTAINING 3-POINT POSITION

Poor: Client cannot maintain 3-pt. position long enough to hit ball.

Inadequate: Client maintains 3-pt. position momentarily to hit ball; occasionally loses balance and uses 4-pt. position for support or sits back.

Optimal: Client has no difficulty maintaining 3-pt. position to hit ball.

Note: If asymmetry is observed, check left or right and score the poorest response on Profile.

C-11. ASYMMETRICAL TONIC NECK PATTERN

Poor: Extreme flexion in support arm when face is turned away; client may lose balance and collapse to ground.

Inadequate: Maintains slight flexion or occasionally extreme flexion in arm on skull side (Fig. 14).

Optimal: Maintains arm extension on skull side.

Note: If asymmetry is observed, check left or right (the side to which head is turned when arm flexion occurs) and score the poorest response on Profile.

C-12. SHOULDER CONTROL

Observe during phases of 3-pt. balance.

Poor: Client cannot maintain cocontraction of shoulder girdle (sags).

Inadequate: Client has difficulty with cocontraction and is unstable on his or her support arm. Tremors may be observed (Fig. 15, 16).

Optimal: Client maintains cocontraction of shoulder girdle and has good stability of the support arm.

Note: If asymmetry is observed, check left or right and score the poorest response on Profile.

C-13. EYE-HAND COORDINATION

Poor: Client is unable to hit ball.

Inadequate: Client makes occasional contact with ball.

Optimal: Client hits ball consistently.

Note: If asymmetry is observed, check left or right and score the poorest response on Profile.

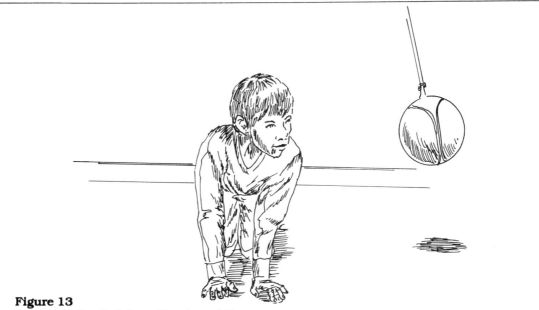

Figure 13
Task: Bat the Ball from Hands and Knees
Scoring
C-1.   Maintains 4-Pt. Position: Score (4)
C-8.   Hand Position of Support Arm: c. Palms Only, score (1)

Comment: Notice that the child's left arm is placed in a locked position, and the shoulder is dropping, indicating decreased stability.

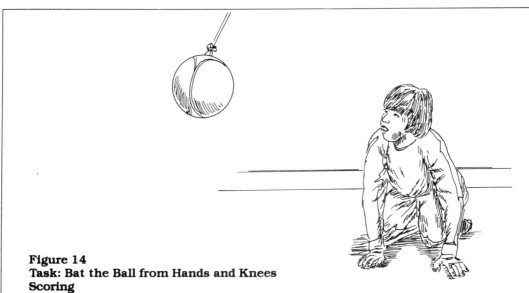

Figure 14
Task: Bat the Ball from Hands and Knees
Scoring
C-1.   Maintains 4-Pt. Position: Score (1) cannot maintain quadruped, sits back on heels
C-6.   Head Righting: Score (1) head remains tilted back in extension
C-7.   Symmetrical Tonic Neck: Score (1) subject sits back on heels
C-11. Asymmetrical Tonic Neck: Score (2) maintains slight flexion in arm on skull side
        (check right)

Comment: As the child's head lifts up to follow the ball, he goes into hip flexion with his weight shifted back. Also note the increased flexor tone on the skull side of the turned head. Notice the wide base of support at the knees.

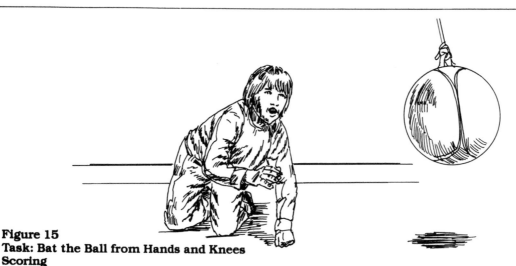

Figure 15
Task: Bat the Ball from Hands and Knees
Scoring
C-1. Maintains 4-Pt. Position: Score (2) maintains momentarily
C-2. Eye Tracking: Score (1) cannot follow visually
C-4. Crosses Midline Visually: Score (1) tilts body
C-5. Crosses Midline Motorically: Score (1) tilts body
C-7. Symmetrical Tonic Neck: Score (2) occasionally sits back
C-8. Hand Position of Support Arm: a. Fisted, score (1)

Comment: Compensatory patterns for stabilization in the upper extremities often require a neutral wrist position since wrist extension sometimes acts to break up a rigid extensor pattern. Notice that the child's entire body turns to the position of the ball, effectively avoiding crossing the midline with his arm.

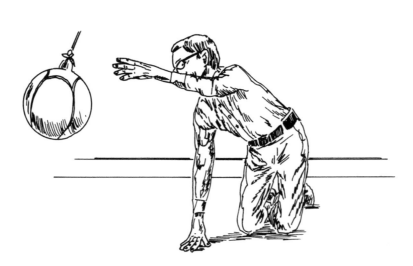

Figure 16
Task: Bat the Ball from Hands and Knees
Scoring
C-5. Crosses Midline Motorically: Score (2) hitting arm crosses midline inconsistently
   because he turns body
C-8. Hand Position of Support Arm: b. Fingertips Only, score (1)
C-12. Shoulder Control: Score (2) unstable on support arm

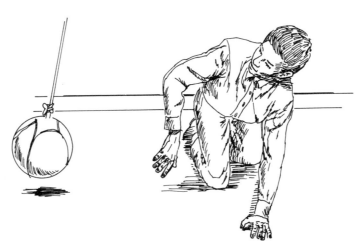

Figure 17
Task: Bat the Ball from Hands and Knees
Scoring
C-5.   Crosses Midline Motorically: Score (1) hits midline out
C-6.   Head Righting: Score (3)
C-7.   Symmetrical Tonic Neck: Score (3) occasionally sits back on heels
C-10. Maintaining 3-Pt. Position: Score (2) occasionally sits back

Comment: This child is hitting the ball from the midline away, rather than across the midline as had been demonstrated.

Client kneels on unstable surface (tiltboard, inverted foam mountain, etc.) and maintains the position while being rocked back and forth slowly. Therapist should also tilt client quickly to observe equilibrium responses.

D-1. ASSUMES KNEELING POSITION
Poor: Requires assistance to get to kneel-standing position (Fig. 18).
Inadequate: Insecure without assistance.
Optimal: Assumes kneeling position independently and with apparent comfort.

D-2. MAINTAINS KNEELING POSITION
(Observe before tilting or rocking.)
Poor: Client cannot maintain kneeling position more than a few seconds (Fig. 19).
Inadequate: Client maintains kneeling position but frequently or easily loses balance.or sits.
Optimal: Client maintains kneeling position (Fig. 21).

D-3. HIP STABILITY
Poor: Hip cocontraction is poor; excessive movement at the hip joints; or rigid and immobile at hip joints [fixed] (Fig. 21).
Inadequate: Able to achieve flexible stability for short periods of time (Fig. 20).
Optimal: Hip cocontraction adequate for stability throughout test, while maintaining flexibility for weight shift.

D-4. TOLERATES MOVEMENT
Poor: Consistently collapses at slight tilt or rock of board (Fig. 19).
Inadequate: When moved, client occasionally sits back on heels or persistently puts hands forward to protect self.
Optimal: Can be rocked while kneeling.

D-5. LATERAL HEAD RIGHTING
Poor: Client's head does not right to vertical when tilted laterally.
Inadequate: Client's head rights inconsistently; head righting is delayed.
Optimal: As body tilts, head rights to vertical immediately.
(Note asymmetry.)

D-6. TRUNK RIGHTING
Poor: As surface is moved quickly, client cannot right trunk adequately and loses balance (Fig. 22).
Inadequate: Client has difficulty with trunk righting, but maintains balance or maintains balance when tilted to one side only.
Optimal: As surface is tilted, client rights trunk to vertical and maintains balance to both sides.
(Note asymmetry.)

D-7. EXTREMITY RIGHTING
Poor: As surface is moved, the arm and/or leg on the high side of the tilt show no sign of response.
Inadequate: Incomplete response or response limited to one extremity or to one side of the body.
Optimal: The arm and/or leg on the high side of the tilt extend and abduct to maintain equilibrium during the tilt (Fig. 22).
Note: If asymmetry is observed, check left or right and score the poorest response on the Profile.

D-8. PROTECTIVE EXTENSION
(Observed during lateral tilt.)
Poor: As surface is moved, the upper extremity on lower side of tilt fails to extend and abduct in a protective response (with support tone) (Fig. 20).
Inadequate: Incomplete or delayed response of upper extremity.
Optimal: Upper extremity on lower side of tilt abducts and extends (with support tone) immediately (Fig. 22) and consistently.
Note: If asymmetry is observed, check left or right and score poorest reponse on the Profile.

D-9. BODY ROTATION

Poor: Trunk rotation is not evident, rigid trunk posture (Fig. 21).

Inadequate: Client maintains rigid trunk posture, but rotational movement occurs occasionally (Fig. 20).

Optimal: Client's trunk remains flexible and rotation is evident with weight shift.

D-10. ANTIGRAVITY EXTENSION

(Client is directed to look down at knees and to remain kneeling.)

Poor: Client collapses in flexion.

Inadequate: Client exhibits increased flexor tone when head is flexed (shoulders, trunk, and hips) (Fig. 20).

Optimal: Client maintains adequate extensor tone throughout the task.

D-11. ANTIGRAVITY FLEXION

(Client is directed to look up at ceiling and to remain kneeling.)

Poor: Shoulders retract and hips hyperextend (lordotic posture) when head tilts back.

Inadequate: Some increase in extension evident either at hips, shoulders, or both.

Optimal: No significant increase in extensor tone is evident.

D-12. SYMMETRICAL TONIC NECK PATTERN

Poor: Client flexes hips and sits back on heels as he looks to the ceiling.

Inadequate: Some increase in flexion evident at hips.

Optimal: No significant increase in hip flexion.

D-13. ASYMMETRICAL TONIC NECK PATTERN (ATNR)

(Client is directed to look to each side.)

Poor: Arms assume ATNR posture as client rotates head (check whether head is facing left or right).

Inadequate: ATNR posture present to one side only; or posture in arms changes in mild response.

Optimal: ATNR posture is not evident.

Note: If asymmetry is observed, check whether left or right direction of face when response noted and score the lowest response on the Profile.

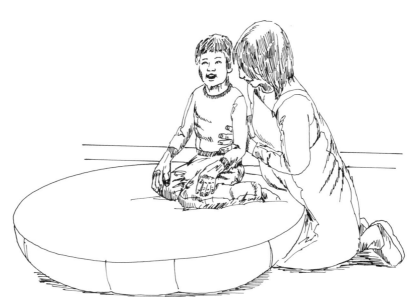

Figure 18
Task: Kneeling Balance
Scoring
D-1.　Assumes Kneeling: Score (1) poor, requires assistance

Comment: On the kneeling task, it is necessary to determine whether the child can assume and/or maintain a kneel standing position. If the child is unable to assume the position, assistance is given to evaluate whether or not he can hold the position.

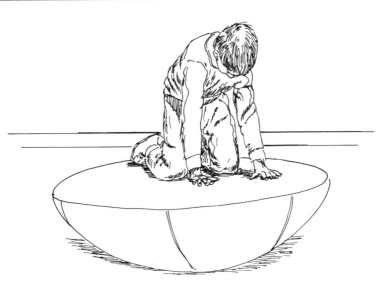

Figure 19
Task: Kneeling Balance
Scoring
D-2.　Maintains Kneeling Position: Score (1) cannot maintain more than a few seconds
D-4.　Tolerates Movement: Score (1) consistently collapses at slight tilt

Comment: As the child loses balance, evaluate protective extension and head righting.

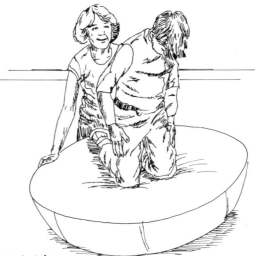

Figure 20
Task: Kneeling Balance
Scoring
D-2. Maintains Kneeling Position:
      Score (2) frequently loses balance
D-3. Hip Stability: Score (3)
D-5. Lateral Head Righting: Score (1) head does not right
D-6. Trunk Righting: Score (3) has difficulty, but maintains balance
D-7. Extremity Righting: Score (2) lower extremity takes some weight, but it is brief
      and the quality poor
D-8. Protective Extension: Score (1) no sign of response
D-9. Body Rotation: Score (3) some rotation evident
D-10. Anti-Gravity Extension: Score (2) flexion-hips

Comment: The child is asked to look up at the ceiling and down at his knees while the
therapist evaluates any changes in postural control that might occur. This child has difficulty
maintaining extensor posture while his head is flexed.

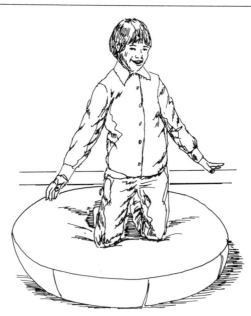

Figure 21
Task: Kneeling Balance
Scoring
D-3. Hip Stability: Score (1) hips rigid and immobile
D-9. Body Rotation: Score (1) rigid trunk posture

Comment: Normally, a small amount of hip flexion and trunk rotation should be maintained
to make the necessary postural adjustments on this surface. This child's locked hips and
pelvis will interfere with his ability to weight shift and to make the appropriate postural
adjustments.

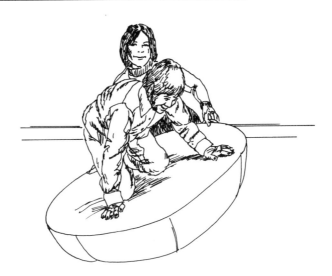

Figure 22
Task: Kneeling Balance
Scoring
D-6.   Trunk Righting: Score (1) loses balance
D-7.   Extremity Righting: Score (5)
D-8.   Protective Extension: Score (5)

Comment: As the child loses balance, he is scored according to the support tone evident in the extremities on the down side of the tilt, the compensatory extension of extremities on the high side, and head righting reactions.

Place ten small pellets or candies in a horizontal row across the midline of the client. Have the client pick up the pellets, one at a time, starting on the far left and drop them in a bottle which has an opening of 1/2" to 3/4" diameter. Then have the client dump pellets out of the bottle. Repeat with client picking up pellets starting on the far right.

E-1. TRUNK STABILITY

Poor: Client loses balance in chair or needs to hold on to or lean on table or chair (Fig. 23, 24, 25).

Inadequate: Client adjusts posture often.

Optimal: Client appears secure in sitting position in chair.

E-2. TRUNK POSTURE

Poor: Shoulder girdle or back unusually rounded and/or hips are flexed more than 100 degrees (Fig. 23, 24).

Inadequate: Occasionally assumes flexed pattern.

Optimal: Back in extension and hips remain at or near 90 degrees of flexion (Fig. 26).

E-3. HEAD POSITION

a. MID-POSITION

Poor: Client's head consistently rotates or tilts to one side (Fig. 23). (Check whether head is facing left or right.)

Inadequate: Client's head occasionally tilts or rotates to one side.

Optimal: Client's head remains in the mid-position (Fig. 26).

b. FLEXED

Poor: Client rests head on table or props head with hand (Fig. 24).

Inadequate: Client flexes neck so eyes are close to table but head is off the table surface (Fig. 25).

Optimal: Client's neck flexes slightly (Fig. 26).

c. EXTENDED

Poor: Client tilts head back past natural position (neck hyperextended).

Inadequate: Client tilts head back past neutral occasionally.

Optimal: Client never tilts head back past neutral.

Scoring instruction: "Mid-position" score in 'ATNR'; "Flexed" score in 'anti-gravity extension'; "Extended" score in 'anti-gravity flexion'; place lowest score in the other open boxes on the Profile.

E-4. USES UNILATERAL REACH

Poor: Client's approach to pellet is scooping action with one or both hands; client then corrals and surrounds a pellet or may accidentally push it out of reach.

Inadequate: Uses unilateral reach occasionally or inaccurately.

Optimal: Hand is directed so that it comes to rest directly on the pellet (Fig. 23, 24, 25, 26).

E-5. GRASP ADEQUATE FOR AGE

Poor: Patterns a through e (below) for children older than 15 months.

Inadequate: Client uses two or more grasp patterns during testing, one of which is forefinger pinch.

Optimal: Pattern f.

a. PALMAR GRASP: Client brings pronated palm down on pellet with thumb in opposition to fingers, especially first three digits (Fig. 23).

b. SUPERIOR PALMAR GRASP: Pellet grasped with thumb and first two fingers, but held against palm for security.

c. LATERAL PINCH (Scissors grasp): Successful prehension between thumb and side of curved index finger.

d. INFERIOR PINCER GRASP: Pellet held between thumb and tip of forefinger and/or middle fingers. Pellet is free of palm but hand rests on table.

e. RADIAL-DIGITAL PINCH: Pellet held between thumb and first and second finger [3-jaw chuck] (Fig. 26).

f. FOREFINGER PINCH: Pellet pinched between thumb and tip of index (or middle) finger. Hand elevated above table surface and accurate overhand grasp used (Fig. 24, 25).

E-6. MOUTHS OR BANGS BOTTLE
Poor: Client's primary behavior with bottle is mouthing or banging it.
Inadequate: Mouths or bangs bottle at least once.
Optimal: No noticeable tendency to mouth or bang bottle.

E-7. AVOIDING REACTIONS
Poor: Excessive abduction of fingers, withdrawal or dorsiflexion of hand when approaching or touching pellets.
Inadequate: Tendency to over-release and/or abduct when releasing the pellets.
Optimal: Graded approach, grip, and release of pellets.

E-8. PUTS PELLETS IN BOTTLE
Poor: Unable to put pellet in bottle.
Inadequate: Has difficulty putting pellet in bottle.
Optimal: Puts pellet in bottle with no difficulty.

E-9. PICKS PELLETS UP IN SEQUENCE
Poor: No consistent sequence in picking up pellets (Fig. 23, 25). (Ask/demonstrate client to pick up pellets in sequence.)
Inadequate: Client picks up pellets consecutively, but does not start at the beginning of row.
Optimal: Client begins at end of row and picks up pellets consecutively.

E-10. CHANGES HAND AT MID-LINE
Poor: Client uses right hand when picking up pellets on the right of body and left hand for pellets on the left side (Fig. 24, 25).
Inadequate: Client does not use one hand consistently.
Optimal: Client uses the same hand consistently for either direction and across mid-line.

E-11. PREFERRED HAND USAGE
Poor: Client does not use one hand consistently; may use left hand when starting with pellets on left, and right hand when starting with pellets on right (Fig. 24, 25).
Inadequate: Predominantly, though not exclusively, uses one hand.
Optimal: Uses dominant hand consistently regardless of starting point.
Note left or right on the profile.

E-12. DUMPS PELLETS OUT
Poor: Unable to dump pellets out of bottle.
Inadequate: Dumps pellets accidentally or after several tries.
Optimal: Intentionally dumps all pellets out of bottle.

E-13. TREMOR
Poor: Pronounced choreoathetoid movements of hand are noticeable during task.
Inadequate: Slight choreoathetoid movements noticeable.
Optimal: Tremor not evident.

E-14. ASSOCIATED MOVEMENTS
Poor: Movement of body parts not essential to the completion of task is evident.
Inadequate: Extraneous movement is minimal or occasional.
Optimal: Extraneous movement is not observable.

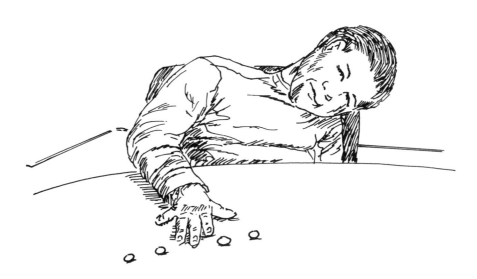

Figure 23
Task: Pellets in Bottle
Scoring
E-1. Trunk Stability: Score (1) needs to hold onto and lean back on chair
E-2. Trunk Posture: Score (1) shoulder girdle and back unusually rounded
E-3. Head Position: a. Mid Position, score (1) head consistently tilts to one side
E-4. Uses Unilateral Reach: Score (5)
E-5. Grasp Adequate for Age: Score (1) uses pattern a. Palmar Grasp on pellet

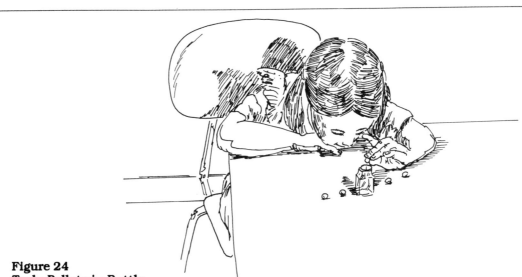

Figure 24
Task: Pellets in Bottle
Scoring
E-1. Trunk Stability: Score (1) leans on table
E-2. Trunk Posture: Score (1) shoulders rounded
E-3. Head Position: a. Mid-Position, score (5); b. Flexed, score (1) head rests on table

Comment: Although this child is pinching the pellet between thumb and second finger, this is a fine fingertip pinch. It is common for Downs Syndrome children to use their middle finger rather than their index finger for pinching tasks. In order to get a good evaluation of trunk stability and sitting, it is important that the child is seated on a chair and at a table of appropriate height.

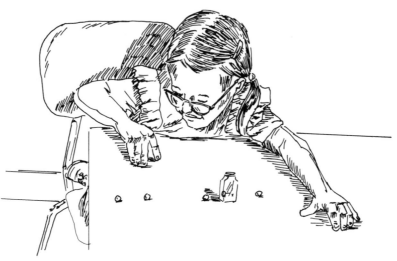

Figure 25
Task: Pellets in Bottle
Scoring
E-1.   Trunk Stability: Score (1) holds/leans on table
E-3.   Head Position: a. Mid-Position, score (3) rotates; b. Flexed, score (3) eyes
         close to table
E-5.   Grasp Adequate for Age: Score (5)
E-9.   Picks Up Pellets in Sequence: Score (1) no sequence
E-10. Changes Hands at Midline: Score (1)
E-11. Preferred·Hand Usage: Score (1) inconsistent (see Fig. 24)

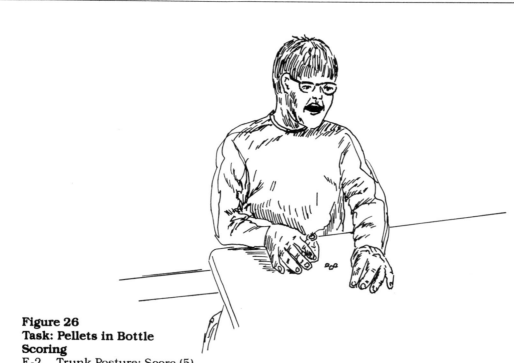

Figure 26
Task: Pellets in Bottle
Scoring
E-2.   Trunk Posture: Score (5)
E-3:   Head Position: a. Mid-Position, score (5); b. Flexed, score (5)
E-5.   Grasp Adequate for Age: Score (1) uses pattern e. Radial-Digital Pinch tograsp pellet

Seat the client in a stable chair with his feet touching the floor. The writing surface should be level with the client's sternum. Place pencil and paper in front of (center) the client. Encourage him to pick up the pencil and draw or scribble.

F-1. TRUNK STABILITY
Poor: Client loses balance in chair or needs to hang on to or lean on table or chair (Fig. 27, 29, 30).
Inadequate: Client needs to adjust posture often.
Optimal: Client appears secure in sitting position in chair (Fig. 28, 34).

F-2. TRUNK POSTURE
Poor: Shoulder girdle or back unusually rounded and/or hips are flexed to more than 100 degrees (Fig. 27, 29, 30, 32, 33).
Inadequate: Occasionally assumes flexed pattern.
Optimal: Back is in extension and hips remain at or near 90 degrees of flexion.

F-3. HEAD POSITION
a. MID-POSITION
Poor: Client's head consistently rotates or tilts to one side (Fig. 27). (Check whether head is facing right or left.)
Inadequate: Client's head occasionally rotates or tilts to one side.
Optimal: Client's head remains in the mid-position (Fig. 28, 30, 31, 33).

b. FLEXED
Poor: Client's head rests on the table or props head with hand (Fig. 27).
Inadequate: Client flexes neck so eyes are close to paper, but head is off the table surface (Fig. 30, 32).
Optimal: Client's neck flexes slightly (Fig. 28, 31, 33).

c. EXTENDED
Poor: Client tilts head back past neutral position.
Inadequate: Client tilts head back past neutral occasionally.
Optimal: Client never tilts head back past neutral.

Scoring instruction: Mid-position score in under ATNR; Flexed score in Anti-Gravity `Extension; Extended score in Anti-Gravity Flexion. Place lowest score in other open boxes on Profile.

F-4. DIFFERENTIATES ENDS OF PENCIL
Poor: Client attempts to draw with either end of pencil indiscriminately.
Inadequate: Client experiments to discover which end works.
Optimal: Client immediately places lead down to draw or scribble.

F-5. POSITIONS PAPER TO CENTER
Poor: Client immediately moves paper to either right or left side or changes position of body so that paper is to one side (Fig. 32, 33). (Check which side of the body is being avoided.)
Inadequate: Client leaves paper in mid-line initially but gradually repositions it or gradually repositions body.
Optimal: Client leaves paper directly in front of body and works with it there.

F-6. USES ONE HAND TO STABILIZE
Poor: Client makes little or no attempt to secure the paper with the empty hand.
Inadequate: Client occasionally uses the empty hand or attempts to use it and/or has difficulty stabilizing the paper.
Optimal: Client uses the empty hand to keep the paper secure and immobile.

F-7. PENCIL POSITION
Poor: a, b, c, or d.
Inadequate: Patterns a,b,c, or d are used intermittently with pattern e (thumb and forefinger opposition).
Optimal: Pattern e.
Note type of pinch:
a. GROSS GRASP: Client holds pencil in palm of hand with fingers and thumb

fisted around it (Fig. 31).

b. LATERAL PINCH: Client holds pencil between the thumb and forefinger with the thumb perpendicular to the forefinger and opposing side of the forefinger rather than tip (pencil may or may not rest on second finger) (Fig. 30, 32, 34).

c. RADIAL-DIGITAL PINCH: Client holds pencil between thumb and first two fingertips (thumb doesn't rest on second finger but opposes it and the forefinger) (Fig. 33).

d. AVOIDS FINGERTIPS ON PENCIL: Any position in which the client does not place any fingertips on the pencil (Fig. 28). (May be a sign of tactile defensiveness.)

e. THUMB AND FOREFINGER OPPOSITION: Pencil is held between the thumb tip and forefinger tip, resting on the distal phalanx of the second finger (Fig. 27).

F-8. FOREARM POSITION
Poor : Palm of drawing hand is parallel to the paper (pronated) (Fig. 28, 29, 31, 34).
Inadequate: Occasionally reverts to pronated position or uses position between pronated and neutral.
Optimal: Ulnar side of arm rests on or is turned toward the paper, and the thumb side is in neutral or slightly rotated toward paper (Fig. 27).

F-9. GRIP STRENGTH
a. HYPOTONIC
Poor: Client can't maintain grip on pencil or may avoid grasping or holding it.
Inadequate: Client has difficulty maintaining grip on pencil and may drop it occasionally.

b. HYPERTONIC
Poor: Client grasps pencil so tightly that knuckles whiten and appear rigid (Fig. 29, 31, 34).
Inadequate: Client's pencil grasp occasionally appears to be tight.
Note: Check if hypotonic or hypertonic and score the poorest response on the Profile.

Optimal: Client's pencil grasp appears firm but flexible, with no sign of rigidity.

F-10. DRAWING PRESSURE
a. HEAVY
Poor: Pencil lead breaks; strokes tear paper; lines are heavy and/or thick (Fig. 29, 34).
Inadequate: Lines vary between heavy and medium visibility.

b. LIGHT
Poor: Pencil marks are thin and difficult to see.
Inadequate: Lines vary between light and medium visibility.
Note: Check if pressure is heavy or light and score the poorest response.
Optimal: Lines are consistently of medium visibility .

F-11. PREFERRED HAND
(Check which hand the client uses primarily for drawing. Observe throughout task.)
a. SWITCHES
Poor: Client uses both hands almost equally (Fig. 30, 32).
Inadequate: Client uses pencil in nondominant hand at some time during the testing.
Optimal: Client does not switch hands.

b. DRAWS ACROSS BODY MID-LINE
(Ask Client to draw a horizontal line from one side of paper to the other.)
Poor: Client turns trunk (Fig. 32), positions paper to one side (Fig. 33), or starts at mid-line of body rather than crossing body with arm. (Fig. 34) (Check which body side client avoids.)
Inadequate: Client turns trunk slightly or leans to one side.
Optimal: Client draws a line from one side of the paper to the other by reaching across the body.
Scoring Instructions: Score lowest response in the open boxes on Profile.

F-12. IMITATES STROKES
(Examiner demonstrates vertical and circular strokes.)
Poor: Patterns c and d.
Inadequate: Attempts patterns a and b.
Optimal: Patterns a and b.

a. VERTICAL: Client draws a vertical line after watching therapist draws one.

b. CIRCULAR: Client draws circular scribbles after watching therapist draw them.

c. SCRIBBLES ONLY: Client merely performs random scribbling motions [does not imitate strokes, copy shapes, or draw] (Fig. 29, 31, 34).

d. BANGS/MOUTHS PENCIL: Client frequently mouths or bangs pencil during activity.

F-13. COPIES CIRCLE/CROSS

a. Show client a circle approximately 4 inches in diameter and ask the client to reproduce it.
Poor: Client does not draw a circle, may scribble with a circular stroke.
Inadequate: Client's reproduction is rough, but recognizable.
Optimal: Client looks at circle and reproduces shape (any size).

b. Show client a cross (with intersecting lines that are 4 inches long) and ask the client to reproduce it.
Poor: Client is unable to copy cross or lines do not intersect.
Inadequate: Reproduction is not accurate, but the lines intersect.
Optimal: Client looks at and reproduces vertical and horizontal intersecting lines (any size).
Scoring Instruction: Score lowest response in the open boxes on Profile.

F-14. UPPER EXTREMITY MOVEMENT

(Observe during imitation and copying, items F-11, F-12, and F-13.)

a. SHOULDER
Poor: Drawing/scribbling movements are directed from the shoulder during most pencil activities; forearm, wrist and/or hand may be completely off the writing surface (Fig. 27, 28, 31, 33).
Inadequate: Drawing movements occasionally come from the shoulder.
Optimal: Movements are primarily controlled by wrist and fingers (no shoulder elevation noted).

b. ELBOW/FOREARM
Poor: Drawing/scribbling movements are directed primarily by the forearm [hand moves off the writing surface in some cases] (Fig. 29, 34).
Inadequate: Movements are frequently, but not primarily, directed by the forearm.
Optimal: Movements are primarily controlled by wrist and fingers.

c. WRIST/FINGER
Poor: Movements are primarily controlled by shoulder or forearm.
Inadequate: Movements are directed by wrist/fingers some of the time (Fig. 30, 32).
Optimal: Drawing/scribbling movements directed by wrist and fingers most of the time.

F-15. ASSOCIATED MOVEMENTS
Poor: Extraneous, nonessential movements are obvious during entire task (watch face and mouth.)
Inadequate: Occasional extraneous movements.
Optimal: No observable extraneous movements.

F-16. TREMOR
Poor: Pronounced choreoathetoid movements of hand or fingers during drawing.
Inadequate: Slight choreoathetoid movements are evident.
Optimal: No tremor evident.

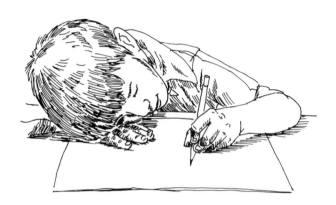

Figure 27
Task: Pencil/Paper Task
Scoring
F-1. Trunk Stability: Score (1) needs to lean on table
F-2. Trunk Posture: Score (1) shoulder girdle and back unusually rounded
F-3. Head Position: a. Mid-Position, score (1) head tilts to one side; b. Flexed, score (1) head rests on table
F-14. Upper Extremity Movement: Score (1) check a.Movement directed from shoulder

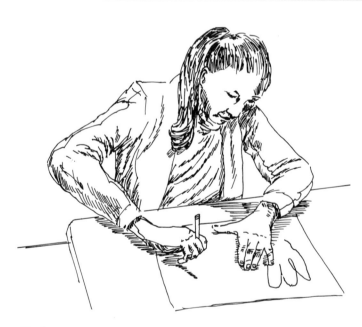

Figure 28
Task: Pencil/Paper Task
Scoring
F-7. Pencil Position: Score (1) d. Avoids Fingertips on Pencil
F-8. Forearm Position: Score (1) forearm pronated
F-14. Upper Extremity Movement: Score (1) check a. Movement directed from shoulder

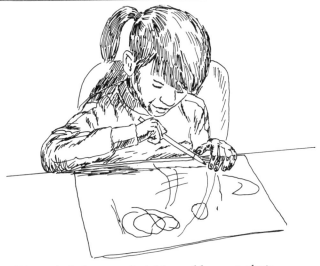

Figure 29
Task: Pencil/Paper Task
Scoring
F-1.   Trunk Stability: Score (1) needs to hang onto table and lean on chair
F-2.   Trunk Posture: Score (1) back unusually rounded
F-7.   Pencil Position: Score (1) check d. Avoids Fingertips on Pencil
F-8.   Forearm Position: Score (1) pronated
F-10. Drawing Pressure: Score (1) check Heavy Lines
F-12. Imitates Strokes: Score (1) check c. Scribbles Only
F-14: Upper Extremity Movement: Score (1) check b. Elbow/Forearm

Comment: Children with poor postural stability sometimes compensate by keeping their arms tucked in close to their body.

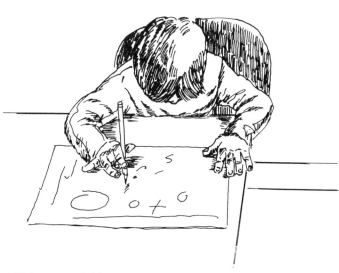

Figure 30
Task: Pencil/Paper Task
Scoring
F-1.   Trunk Stability: Score (1) leans on table
F-2.   Trunk Posture: Score (1) rounded
F-3.   Head Position: a. Mid-Position, score (5); b. Flexed, score (3)
F-7.   Pencil Position: Score (1) check b. Lateral Pinch
F-8.   Forearm Position: Score (1) pronated
F-14. Upper Extremity Movement: Score (5) movements directed primarily from wrist and fingers

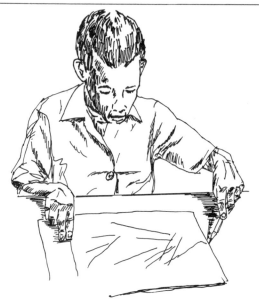

Figure 31
Task: Pencil/Paper Task
Scoring
F-6.   Uses One Hand to Stabilize: Score (2) has difficulty stabilizing paper
F-7.   Pencil Position: Score (1) check a. Gross Grasp
F-8.   Forearm Position: Score (1) palm parallel to table surface
F-12. Imitates Strokes: Score (1) check c. Scribbles Only
F-14. Upper Extremity Movement: Score (1) check a. Movement primarily by shoulder
F-15. Associated Movements: Score (1) extraneous movements of mouth, tongue, and jaw,

Comment: Notice the overflow movements in the mouth and jaw.

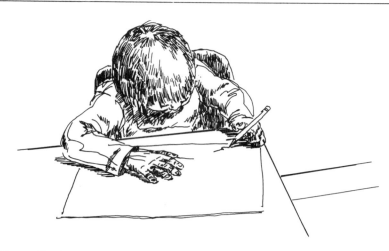

Figure 32
Task: Pencil/Paper Task
Scoring
F-2.   Trunk Posture: Score (2) occasionally assumes flexed pattern
F-3.   Head Position: a. Mid-Position, score (1) check left; b. Flexed, score (2)
F-5.   Positions Paper to Center: Score (1) turns body
F-7.   Pencil Position: Score (1) check b. Lateral Pinch
F-11. Preferred Hand: Score (1) check b. Draws across Body Midline, turns trunk
F-14. Upper Extremity Movement: Score (3) check c. Wrist/Finger,

Comment: Notice the trunk rotated in the direction of the task which avoids the necessity to cross the midline.

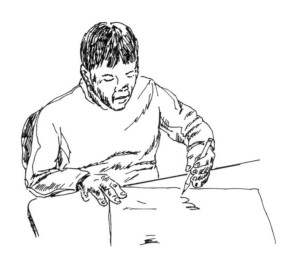

Figure 33
Task: Pencil/Paper Task
Scoring
F-2.   Trunk Posture: Score (2) rounded low back
F-3.   Head Position: a. Mid-Position, score (5); b. Flexed, score (5) neck flexed slightly
F-5.   Positions Paper to Center: Score (1) moves paper to left body space
F-7.   Pencil Position: Score (1) check c. Radial-Digital Pinch
F-14. Upper Extremity Movement: Score (1) check a. movements directed primarily
         from shoulders

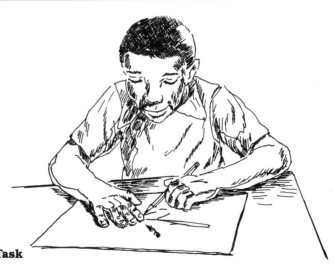

Figure 34
Task: Pencil/Paper Task
Scoring
F-7.   Pencil Position: Score (1) check b. Lateral Pinch
F-8.   Forearm Position: Score (1), palm pronated
F-9.   Grip Strength: Score (1) check b. Hypertonic, grasps tightly
F-10. Drawing Pressure: Score (1) check a. Heavy, lines heavy and thick
F-11. Preferred Hand: Score (1) check b. Draws Across Body Midline
F-12. Imitates Strokes: Score (1) check c. Scribbles Only
F-14. Upper Extremity Movement: Score (1) check b. Elbow/Forearm primarily

Comment: Notice how stress and tension are communicated by shoulder elevation and
heavy, darkly drawn lines.

Place paper and primary scissors in front of client. Ask client to cut (any way he can). After client demonstrates ability to use scissors, ask him to cut along a 1/4 inch wide straight line and then along a curved line (a blunt-edged marking pen makes a 1/4 inch wide line).

G-1. TRUNK STABILITY

Poor: Client loses balance in chair or needs to hold on to or lean on table or chair.

Inadequate: Client adjusts posture often.

Optimal: Client appears secure in sitting position in chair (Fig. 36).

G-2. TRUNK POSTURE

Poor: Shoulder girdle or back is unusually rounded and/or hips are flexed to more than 100 degrees.

Inadequate: Occasionally assumes flexed pattern.

Optimal: Back is in extension and hips remain at or near 90 degrees of flexion.

G-3. HEAD POSITION

a. MID-POSITION

Poor: Head tilts or rotates to one side (Fig 35). Note which side.

Inadequate: Head tilts or rotates to one side occasionally.

Optimal: Head in mid-position (Fig. 36).

b. FLEXED

Poor: Overly-flexed with chin on chest, or head supported on table or hands.

Inadequate: Occasionally rests chin on chest or supports head on table or hands.

Optimal: Head slightly flexed for eye-hand coordination (Fig. 36).

c. EXTENDED

Poor: Client tilts head back past neutral position.

Inadequate: Client tilts head back past neutral occasionally.

Optimal: Client never tilts head back past neutral.

Scoring Instruction: Mid-position score in ATNR; Flexed score in Anti-Gravity Extension; Extended score in Anti-Gravity Flexion. Place lowest score in other open boxes on the Profile.

G-4. SHOULDER POSITION

Poor: Shoulders elevated (fixated) and/or arms elevated to shoulder height (Fig. 35).

Inadequate: Excessive shoulder movement or occasional shoulder elevation during cutting.

Optimal: Shoulders relaxed and at appropriate height during cutting task (Fig. 36).

G-5. FOREARM HOLDING PAPER

a. PRONATED

Poor: Arm pronated so palm is parallel to floor (Fig. 35).

Inadequate: Forearm partially pronated.

b. SUPINATED

Poor: Arm supinated so palm faces ceiling.

Inadequate: Forearm partially supinated.

Optimal: Client holds paper with forearm in neutral with thumb up and ulnar side down (Fig.36).

G-6. HAND GRIP HOLDING PAPER

a. HYPOTONIC

Poor: Grip weak, drops paper easily.

Inadequate: Grasp hypotonic, but adequate to hold paper.

b. HYPERTONIC

Poor: Grip overly tense or tight; paper crumples.

Inadequate: Occasionally grips paper too tightly.

Optimal: Securely grasps paper without tension.

G-7. FOREARM CUTTING PAPER

a. PRONATED

Poor: Forearm pronated, palm facing down (Fig. 35).

Inadequate: Occasionally pronates forearm or uses position between pronated and neutral.

b. SUPINATED

Poor: Forearm supinated, palm up.

Inadequate: Supinated occasionally or uses position between supinated and neutral.

Optimal: Forearm in mid-position, thumb up.

G-8. WRIST POSITION DURING CUTTING

Poor: Maintains rigid flexion or extension of the wrist or ulnar deviation (Fig. 35).

Inadequate: Unable to grade flexion and extension for smooth cutting.

Optimal: Wrist in neutral position with dynamic flexion and extension on curved lines.

G-9. HAND CUTTING PAPER

Poor: Patterns a or b on the scissors.

Inadequate: Patterns a or b are used intermittently with pattern c.

Optimal: Pattern c.

a. LATERAL PINCH - Thumb opposes lateral surface of forefinger.

b. FOREFINGER PINCH - Thumb opposes tip of forefinger.

c. THUMB/HAND OPPOSITION - Thumb in one hole of scissor, middle finger in other. Thumb opposes all fingers simultaneously and middle finger directly (Fig. 36).

G-10. UNUSED FINGERS

Poor : Fingers remain extended and/or abducted; or unused fingers flex and extend in gross grasp pattern.

Inadequate: Intermittent or occasional extension or abduction of unused fingers.

Optimal: Unused fingers remain flexed during cutting.

G-11. VISUAL ORIENTING

Poor : Lack of visual attention to task.

Inadequate: Inconsistent visual attention to task.

Optimal: Consistent visual attention to the cutting task.

G-12. CUT IS CONTINUOUS/SMOOTH

Poor: Cut is primarily choppy; each squeeze of scissor is evident; paper is more torn than cut; or client does not have adequate strength/coordination to manipulate scissor to cut sharply.

Inadequate: Cut is occasionally choppy or ragged (Fig. 36).

Optimal: Cut is continuous and smooth.

G-13. STRAIGHT LINE IS ACCURATE

Poor: Cut is either outside the line more than 50 percent of length or more than 1/4 inch outside the line approximately 25 percent of length or more.

Inadequate: Cut is outside, but close to, line for 75 percent of length.

Optimal: Cut is primarily on the 1/4 inch wide straight line.

G-14. CURVED LINE IS ACCURATE

(Same criteria as above.)

G-15. PREFERRED HAND

Poor: Client frequently switches hand while cutting, or client uses hand opposite that used for paper/pencil task.

Inadequate: Client occasionally switches hands while cutting.

Optimal: Client consistently uses the same hand to cut that he used in the paper/pencil task.

Note which hand is used most often.

G-16. TREMOR

Poor: Pronounced choreoathetoid movements are evident during task.

Inadequate: Occasional slight tremor during task.

Optimal: Tremor is not evident.

G-17. ASSOCIATED MOVEMENTS

Poor: Extraneous, non-essential movements are obvious during task (Check face and mouth).

Inadequate: Occasional extraneous movements.

Optimal: No observable non-essential movements.

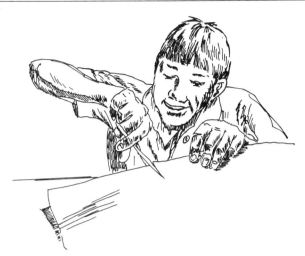

Figure 35
Task: Scissor Task
Scoring

G-3. Head Position: a. Mid-Position, score (1) head rotates to side
G-4. Shoulder Position: Score (1) shoulders and arm elevated and fixed
G-5. Forearm Holding Paper: Score (1) check a. Pronated,
G-7. Forearm Cutting Paper: Score (1) check a. Pronated, forearm cutting paper is so pronated that it is going into internal rotation
G-8. Wrist Position During Cutting: Score (1) wrist in ulnar deviation
G-9. Hand Cutting Paper: Score (5) check c. Thumb/Hand Opposition,

Comment: Regressing to a lower developmental pattern is a common response when a child's sensorimotor abilities are over-stressed. This child has reverted to a pronated approach to the scissor and paper.

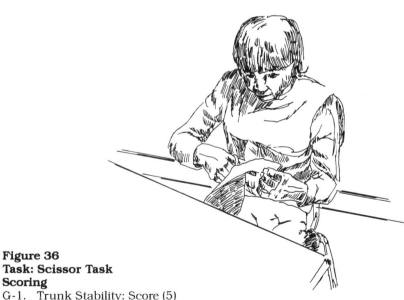

Figure 36
Task: Scissor Task
Scoring

G-1. Trunk Stability: Score (5)
G-3. Head Position: a. Mid-Position, score (5); b. Flexed, score (5)
G-4. Shoulder Position: Score (5)
G-5. Forearm Holding Paper: Score (5)
G-9. Hand Cutting Paper: Score (5)
G-12. Cut Continuous/Smooth: Score (3) cut occasionally choppy

Comment: Note optimal posture and scissor manipulation.